Fighting Covid-19, the Unequal Opportunity Killer:

You are not helpless in the face of the Covid-19 epidemic

Irving A. Cohen, MD, MPH

Fellow of the American College of Preventive Medicine

www.epidemicwall.com

Center for Health Information
Topeka, Kansas
www.centerforhealthinformation.com

Copyright 2021 by Irving A. Cohen, M.D.,M.P.H.

All rights reserved. None of this publication may be reproduced, stored in a retrieval system, resold, redistributed or transmitted in any form or by any means (electronic, mechanical, photocopying, recording or otherwise) without the prior written permission of the publisher.

Published by
Center for Health Information, Inc.
Topeka, KS

Library of Congress Control Number: 2021900447

Cohen, Irving A. 1944-

Fighting Covid-19,
the
Unequal Opportunity Killer:

You are not helpless in the face of the Covid-19 epidemic

ISBN 978-0-9820111-6 4 (Paperback)
ISBN 978-0-9820111-5-7 (E-book)

Editor, Alice Heiserman
Cover Illustrator, Bailey Coon

Printed in the United States of America

Contents

	Introduction		*vii*
Chapter	1	**You Can Fight Back**	1
Chapter	2	**What is Prevention?**	7
Chapter	3	**Wrong Ideas**	17
Chapter	4	**The Inflammatory Spectrum of Diabetes**	39
Chapter	5	**Evaluating Your Own Status**	51
Chapter	6	**Objective Lab Tests**	63
Chapter	7	**Boosting Vitamin D**	79
Chapter	8	**Reversing Insulin Resistance**	85
Chapter	9	**Diets Are Not All The Same**	91
Chapter	10	**Deadly Ingredients**	109
Chapter	11	**Labels, Labels, Labels**	123
Chapter	12	**Starting Out**	141
Chapter	13	**Metabolism Improvement**	151
Chapter	14	**One Day At A Time**	165
	Appendix		177
		Dealing with dietary restrictions	177
		Meal plan suggestions	178
		Starter recipes	182
		Supplements to consider	188
		Avoid chemical flavor-enhancers	192
		Deciding on sweeteners	194
		The fats you eat	197
		Recipe worksheet	200
	About the Author		202

Other Books by Dr. Cohen

Diabetes Recovery:
Reversing Diabetes with the New Hippocratic Diet®
Center for Health Information ISBN 978-0-9820111-0-2

Doctor Cohen's New Hippocratic Diet® Guide:
How to Really Lose Weight and Beat the Obesity Epidemic
Center for Health Information ISBN 978-0-9820111-9-5

La Nueva Dieta Hipocrática™ del Dr. Cohen:
Cómo realmente bajar de peso y vencer la epidemia de la obesidad
Center for Health Information ISBN 978-0-9820111-8-8

Cooking for the New Hippocratic Diet®
Center for Health Information ISBN 978-0-9820111-7-1

Addiction: The High-Low Trap
Health Press ISBN 0-929173-10-4

Introduction

I have dedicated my previous books to a particular group that is suffering. Facing the current Covid-19 epidemic things are different, so this book is dedicated to all of us. Those who are isolated at home, those who are working on the front lines, and those who are just trying to get by. We are all dealing with both the common enemy of a virus and the internal enemy of fear and uncertainty. We can and should take all the necessary steps to protect ourselves and those around us, whether they are our loved ones or total strangers. There is one more thing you can do. Many were exposed and had mild cases while others became severely ill and some died. Once ill, the difference may be their immune system doing what it is supposed to do or simply allowing this terrible illness to tip them over the edge. If you have been told you are in a high risk group, what can you do about it? Are you are older? Do you have a chronic disease? Are you Black, Native American, or Hispanic? Do you live with the others or in a congregate setting?

You are not helpless in the face of the Covid-19 epidemic! You may have options. Put aside learned helplessness and take action. Those unchangeable risk factors, such as race or age, may not be the <u>cause</u> of your high risk. Instead, they are statistical associations because of underlying chronic inflammation in your group, which can be objectively measured by your doctor. It is controllable, and you can begin right now. Whether you will face the need for extra protection from Covid-19 or not, you will also be reversing other conditions that steal years from your life. My experiences in Preventive Medicine and Public Health taught me to help people overcome issues they thought were irreversible. You can do more, strengthen your personal defensive wall, and allow your immune system to fight off attackers. Do it now.

Irving A. Cohen, MD,MPH

Fellow of the American College of Preventive Medicine

Stay Informed

- The purpose of this book is to provide the reader valuable information and opinion during a serious epidemic. Our knowledge of this disease is continually evolving .

- Nothing in this book should be construed as individual medical advice. All readers are urged to obtain medical evaluation and support when needed. The reader should consult his or her own physician for such advice.

- The information presented in this book has been obtained from sources believed to be authentic and reliable. Although great care has been taken to ensure the accuracy of the information presented, the author and the publisher cannot assume responsibility for the validity of all the materials or the consequences for their use.

1

You Can Fight Back

Have you felt helpless as the Covid-19 epidemic suddenly became everyone's dominant concern and fear? The epidemic and its consequences have affected every person globally, whether they were infected or not. Some people were more likely to be infected than others, but the inequality of the disease only begins there. Once infected, why are some people more likely to suffer and possibly to die than others?

What can you do on your own to protect yourself? Vaccines are becoming available and you should take advantage of the opportunity to become vaccinated as soon as you can. The vaccines seem highly effective, but we do not know yet just how long their protection may last. We do know that mutations of the virus have begun to show up and are spreading rapidly. Whether the new vaccines will offer protection from each new mutation is also an unanswered question. Will Covid-19 come back every year, just like influenza, requiring a newer vaccine each time? That too remains to be seen.

What else can you do to add protection? One way, which you are likely already doing, is to hunker down to try to

Chapter 1: You Can Fight Back

prevent becoming infected. Quarantining, isolating, and sanitizing are all legitimate strategies and should be followed as best as possible. The world has quickly learned that even when these strategies are effective, they are highly disruptive. The world has to go on; people have to eat, pay the rent, care for their family, and do many things we had taken for granted before all this began.

Doing all those things—isolating, wearing masks, and washing your hands are all reactive approaches. As physicians and scientists attempt to figure out how to best fight this disease, public officials want to slow it down so that their populations remain healthy and the hospital systems across the world are not overwhelmed. The so-called "flattening-the-curve" strategies are simply stretching out the period until the entire world is exposed, and those who survive develop immunity or have been vaccinated. The truth is that epidemics have come and gone over thousands of years. In each case, they did not just come through once; they reverberated through multiple cycles. Many still exist, although their impact is usually controllable through immunization and medication.

Making the situation seemingly worse is the knowledge that race, age, and pre-existing diseases seem to dictate whether an infected person is likely to recover or die. Yet, grim as this knowledge is, it also gives us hope by showing us clues about how we can harden our defense against this disease. The good news is that the majority of people who are infected will not die. Some lucky ones will have an easier time, not even knowing that they were infected. We call these people *asymptomatic*. Many others will know they are ill and have a rough time. Then, some will become extremely ill, requiring prolonged hospitalization, and some may not make it. We quickly learned that those with certain issues have the roughest time. We also discovered that race and age predict complications, but why is that?

The cause is **inflammation**, your body's response to something that is going wrong. You can see inflammation in the classic redness and swelling of an insect bite or infection. Your body, recognizing that something is wrong, uses inflammation as a defense mechanism to fight the invader or irritant. What you do not see are similar defenses when inflammation is internal. Often, your body overreacts, attacking an imaginary foe as your immune system becomes out of control. We call those events *autoimmune res*ponses or disorders. When your own immune system attacks parts of your body, it creates inflammation, as if you were your own enemy!

Physicians who specialize in rheumatology, allergy, or dermatology all spend a great deal of their work treating such disorders. They may have to resort to powerful medications to quiet an over-reactive immune system. These medicines can be highly effective but weaken your immune system from doing its job to protect you from true dangers. Doctors who specialize in fighting infectious diseases face the opposite problem. People who have a compromised immune system cannot defend themselves well from infections that others can handle.

The worst danger of inflammation can be its hidden nature. Hidden inflammation can happen quite early in chronic disease. Those early chronic conditions are often not recognized enough, either by the sufferers or their doctors.

Chapter 1: You Can Fight Back

Have you known of anyone who thought they were in perfect health yet suddenly died? Many of these so-called "chronic conditions" start years or decades before they become obvious. They do their damage without the victim's knowledge. The good news is you and your physician can learn how early chronic disease creates inflammation, silently attacking your body. *If you're willing to try*, you can reverse these problems. You can do this without new costly medicines, and you may be able to reduce the need for medications you are already using.

What does this inflammatory reaction have to do with the current deadly epidemic? Covid-19 is a viral infection that causes havoc by creating terrible inflammation. It can attack most body organs. If a person's body has a weak spot, someplace where inflammation from a chronic disease is already at work, the combination can be devastating. That is why, those at the highest risk of death or severe debilitating infection are people with such underlying issues. It does not matter whether they know about their chronic disease or not. When this dreaded virus adds its level of inflammation, the combination may be deadly.

The data for severe and deadly outcomes of Covid-19 show the three highest risk factors. Those are **age, race,** and ***known* chronic conditions**. Age and race increase the chances of being exposed to the infection. Age increases the chance of exposure because there is a higher chance of exposure in nursing homes. Race and ethnicity may influence you socio-economic status, determining who works in crowded environments, such as food processing facilities. Crowded public transportation, getting to work in big cities, is an exposure risk factor. Once exposed and infected, age and race play a different role. In the United States, the odds of having a chronic disease that causes inflammation are highest for older people, Blacks and Native-Americans.

The likelihood of dying from Covid-19, particularly if you are Black, is a combination of three factors. The risk of exposure, the risk of a severe case of the disease once exposed, and finally, the quality of care if you become ill. All three of these have deep historical social and economic roots; for many they involve historic and ongoing racism, prejudice and injustice. Continue to do all you can about reducing exposure risk and getting the best medical care but do not ignore your risk of severe infection if exposed. Whatever your race or age, improving how your body responds is within your control.

It is in your hands, because you can fight those uneven odds. Experience and the availability of testing have shown us the way. Some infected people face a tremendous battle to survive; others can fight this off more easily. They may have so mild an illness that they have no symptoms at all. There are no guarantees, but defending yourself *before* becoming infected greatly improves your odds. Fighting pre-existing inflammation can help build a wall of protection against both this epidemic and possible future illnesses. Even were there no Covid-19 and no epidemic, the steps you can take will reverse the odds of your developing other diseases in the future.

What are your odds? If you are in a higher-risk group, you should be more concerned, but what if you are not in a high-risk group? Foolishly, some individuals are arrogant and ignore all precautions. Besides the risk of dying themselves, some just get sick enough to pass the Covid-19 virus on and sicken or kill others. The supposed risk factors of age and race only describe an association of factors. No one is immune to the risks of the real underlying issues. Ten years ago, the Centers for Disease Control (CDC) projected that one in three adults could be diabetic by 2050.[1] That is but one of several chronic disease risk factors growing at an alarming rate; yet, they may not always be obvious to the victim. So, while it is true that some underlying issues are found more often in some groups, no one should feel safe because they are not old or not a member of a minority group.

Keep an open mind and consider whether you need to harden your health and build an extra wall to stay well.

---

1. Boyle et al. **Projection of the year 2050 burden of diabetes in the US adult population: dynamic modeling of incidence, mortality, and prediabetes prevalence.** *Population Health Metrics*, 2010,8:29
http://www.pophealthmetrics.com/content/8/1/29

2

What is Prevention?

If you already have high-risk factors, what good is prevention? "Preventive Medicine" is a broad and well-recognized medical specialty, not the simple catch-phrase that marketers use. It is better to *prevent* disease rather than cure it. This idea goes back to ancient times. Some religious practices mentioned in the Old Testament may lead to better health. The ancient Greeks, generations before Hippocrates, worshipped Hygeia, goddess of prevention and good health.

Teaching people how to prevent disease always used to be linked to healing. Calling a healer *"Doctor"* really means a learned teacher. For many years, society looked upon doctors as people who could, hopefully, teach others to remain healthy. Sometimes what they taught was factual and worked; at other times, it was based on superstition and myth.

Preventive Medicine and Public Health, my medical specialty, is a branch of medicine recognized by the American Medical Association for about seven decades. It focuses on the prevention of disease, and it requires years of additional specialized post-graduate education and experience.

Prevention, when effective, is more sensible than

Chapter 2 : What is Prevention?

waiting until illness strikes and attempting to cure a disease. Unfortunately, efforts and money spent on prevention today are a minuscule proportion of the vast amounts spent curing disease. Additionally, some efforts labeled "*prevention*" are ineffective and even harmful. True prevention is rarely a money-maker. So instead, we see major programs and products attempting to promote *panaceas* or *cure-alls* rushing into the market place. These false claims fill a vacuum since the general public understands the common-sense notion that prevention is worthwhile.

The public welcomes preventive measures but has grown weary and skeptical because of false hope from ideas and products that turn out to be hoaxes. In the late 1970s, the Federal government began a massive program to convince Americans that low-fat dieting was good for them. **That action caused the number of people suffering from unwanted weight-gain and type II diabetes to more than double.** Unfortunately, many false prevention ideas caused far more disease than they prevented over the past four decades. Today, chronic disease affects more Americans than ever. In the view of international health experts, we have slipped to 37th place in overall health system rankings,[2] among all the nations of the world .

Take a moment to understand what prevention means and how this relates to the current national health crisis and ultimately to you. Preventive medicine has three unique components. These are called:

---

2. Murray,C et al. **Ranking 37th — Measuring the Performance of the U.S. Health Care System**. *N Engl J Med* 362:98-99 2010;   DOI: 10.1056/NEJMp0910064

Primary Prevention,

Secondary Prevention and

Tertiary Prevention.

Each is needed in the fight against disease and unnecessary death, and they often overlap.

Primary Prevention

Primary prevention means taking some action so that disease or injury should never occur. Primary prevention can be the most powerful tool we have, but only when it is done effectively. Once a preventive measure becomes effective, we sometimes forget the serious reasons it is needed. It is sometimes difficult for people to understand why they should be taking that preventive measure.

A good example is immunization. There is no question that widespread immunization is an effective tool for preventing certain disease outbreaks. People who have already suffered through those disease outbreaks understand its value. However, because immunization may have done such a good job preventing a disease, younger people who never faced the same outbreaks may not see the reason to bother. They are fortunate to lack first-hand knowledge of what occurred without this important preventive measure. When many people recently skipped measles immunization, they caused an epidemic of that disease.

One weakness of primary prevention is that it may be difficult to understand what works and what does not work. In ancient times, lacking the science to provide an understanding

Chapter 2 : What is Prevention?

of the basis for disease, some prevention took the form of superstition. Some superstition was innocent enough when it came to wearing amulets to ward off disease but other actions could do damage when harmful actions were taken to protect the community.

Examples of *Primary prevention* against Covid-19 are the widespread use of masks and other protective equipment, quarantine, and isolation, as well as widespread testing and contact tracing. Done well, and with the understanding and cooperation of the public, they can work well. Done clumsily or stupidly, they can cause a backlash and rejection.

The recent successful vaccine development can become a potent weapon of *primary prevention* against the Covid-19 epidemic, once immunization is in widespread use, confers long-lasting immunity and remains effective despite virus mutation. Keep up with that ever-changing development. This book's focus is teaching you how you can help yourself right now using the next topic, *secondary prevention*.

Secondary Prevention

Secondary prevention for any diseases should mean recognizing problems and intervening at the earliest possible stage. This is not being done early enough today. Instead, as a nation, we wait until people are at a stage where the prescription of medication, hospitalization, or other action can be justified.

What do you expect will happen when the agenda for change is decided by drug makers and food processors' influence? As an example, Type II diabetes is a continuum. It begins years before it reaches the stage where medication is needed. It can be detected at an early point using objective tests and reversed without medication. Instead, we have turned to methods that start with a few dollars of medication a year but rapidly progress as the patient deteriorates. Some people end up on $20,000 of medication a year. Often, they continue to be less healthy than those people who were able to reverse their problems, so that they need little or no medication.

What does this have to do with Covid-19, and how does this affect your risk during the Covid-19 epidemic? Secondary prevention will not change the likelihood of being infected, but secondary prevention may make the difference between having a mild or asymptomatic case and a severe case of the disease. Many people who were infected report feeling ill and getting over it. On the other hand, many people with risk factors were so severely impacted that they spent weeks hospitalized. Which would you prefer?

What are the risk factors? You may have heard that some of these are race, age, and location. That is a half-truth, for it does not explain *why* these are risk factors. **You cannot change your chronological age or your race.** You have to dig two levels deeper to understand them, to get away from the racist and ageist myths that can make people despair. **You will discover that the underlying risk issue is actually inflammation**. Remember, the damage of Covid-19 is done through inflammation. Whatever organ system it attacks, it does so by causing hyper-inflammation. If there is <u>already other inflammation</u> from the chronic disease present, this extra inflammation teams up with it to worsen both conditions.

The chronic disease may be known, or it may still be

Chapter 2 : What is Prevention?

hidden. Many epidemiologists worldwide believe that the true death toll from Covid-19 disease is far more than the official tolls. Without universal testing, when someone with a known chronic condition dies suddenly, it is easy to attribute their death to that known chronic condition. Simultaneously, as the epidemic death tolls have risen, so have death tolls in general. Epidemiologists can compare overall death rates in a location and for a time of year with the expectations based on previous years. What they may see is an excessive number of deaths explained by other causes. It is impossible for them to say with ironclad certainty that it was due to the addition of Covid-19. Some may not be infected but their reason for dying may be because another health problem was ignored or overlooked because of the epidemic. Others may have died because of disruptive financial and social upheaval many are going through. Sadly, the true toll of this horrible disease may be grossly underreported and unrecognized.

Historical factors mean that people in high-risk groups are already more likely to become ill, and once they do become infected, they also face greater danger than others. Consider employment and living conditions for many African-Americans in New York City. Those conditions make the odds of becoming infected high. One of the many reasons is that they are more likely to use crowded public transportation and live in crowded housing. If you are older, you are at risk for congregant living, such as residing in nursing homes and senior care facilities. This closeness also can foster disease transmission once the disease is introduced into such a facility. Those issues may be too powerful to be stopped completely by primary prevention.

Fighting Covid-19, the Unequal Opportunity Killer

When primary prevention is insufficient, secondary prevention becomes the next line of defense. Minority groups in the United States already have higher rates of many chronic issues, such as diabetes and hypertension. Older people in congregate care facilities often already have multiple chronic diseases. When Covid-19 is introduced, serious illness and death rates are greater. **Whether you believe you are in a high-risk group or not, you can begin right now to strengthen your protective wall.**

The wall **you** can build to protect yourself from a more serious illness is to reverse your chronic disease. No, this is not magical thinking. You can do it—what better time than now when it will make such a serious difference. Later, if you maintain these changes, you will benefit in many other ways, but today the aim is to make you stronger in resisting should you become infected with Covid-19.

You may have fought some of these battles, thinking you were doing all the right things. Yet, your problems with blood pressure, weight, and diabetes might have worsened with time. Your doctor could have scolded you and convinced you that something was wrong with you. Just bringing up the subject can make you feel mocked and depressed. The good news is that most of you can succeed. Although you can not change your age or race, using secondary prevention can give you the tools to equalize your risks and level the field. You will learn how to do this—keep reading and know you can triumph.

When your old plan did not work, you did not fail! Your old plan failed you.

Chapter 2 : What is Prevention?

Tertiary Prevention

Tertiary prevention is what we think of as "routine" clinical medicine. When the first two barriers are broken down, this is where the health system attempts to save you. With our health system facing a new challenge from Covid-19, it is learning more about its enemy. Efforts continue to find a better way, a magic drug, or a perfect protocol that allows people to be treated.

Unfortunately, inequities about who gets better care will not be solved on the spot. There is also no way to have a crystal ball to predict the future, despite the abundance of "experts" who pretend to do so. When people reach the point of needing acute medical care, the best care will come from providers who are observant, caring, and open-minded about learning what does and does not work. This is a constantly changing area, where new developments will continue to provide changing methods and perspectives.

This book will provide information about secondary prevention. Continue reading to learn how to build a wall within yourself. You are the one in control. Of course, you need to keep following current recommendations regarding primary prevention, particularly immunization. That is the first wall, and it is very important. Sometimes that first wall will work effectively, but other times it will be breached. When you are exposed to Covid-19, your having already understood and taken measures to protect yourself will matter most.

For those who do become ill, accessibility to and overworked clinical care system may be outside of your control at that point. **Focus on what you can change, and you can strengthen the defenses for yourself and your family.** Put aside the myths and the profit-making lies you have become accustomed to hearing. Be open so that you can learn new ways that benefit you, not some distant corporation or industry lobby.

Chapter 3

Wrong Ideas

"The greatest discovery of my generation is that human beings can alter their lives by altering their attitudes of mind."

William James
(1842-1910, The Father of American Psychology)

Wrong ideas can kill you. This, of course, was true even before the current health crisis. Newspaper articles, media coverage, and internet blogs are full of planted information, supplied by publicists working for those who gain financially from these wrong ideas. Misinformation is so widespread that those writing the articles may not understand they are being manipulated. Having unbiased information can allow you to prevent those chronic diseases that cause inflammation. That can save your life. Both the chronic disease itself and the increased susceptibility to Covid-19 put you in danger. You must first learn what tainted advice is, even when you have followed it for years. Sometimes false knowledge is totally wrong; other times, it is partially true but twisted and overplayed.

It would be great if education in health knowledge alone were the key to getting healthy. That might be true *if* all health advice were true, honest, effective, and applied equally to

Chapter 3: Wrong Ideas

everyone.

If it were, then politics would not be involved.

If it were, then the test of a health campaign would be whether it actually improved the health of those receiving it.

If it were, it would be free of commercial interests.

If it were, scientists would always openly reveal financial or career incentives associated with their interpretation of science.

If it were, broadcast and print media would actually read the studies themselves before publicizing them, instead of using someone else's press release about the study.

Bad information can be twisted to wrong ends. Those manipulating information take advantage of our quest to stay healthy. People are not stupid; we do <u>try</u> to do the right thing. When the results are bad, we become disillusioned and stop trying. Many of us join a gym in January, thinking we will magically lose weight and become fit. Often, we quit by February, stuck for a full year's dues. Other times, we follow the fad of the day, whether it is dietary, magical supplements, or some other plan. We often blame ourselves when we are unable to achieve our desired goal. Sometimes we seek prescriptions that do not resolve our problems, only add more ineffective treatments as things become worse.

Wake up! In the fable "The Emperor's New Clothes," it takes a child to state what everyone is capable of seeing but is afraid to say. The question to ask yourself is, "am I doing the right thing?" If you think you are, but it is not effective, is it truly the right thing?

In the 1970s, an actress made millions by exhorting people to buy her videotapes and do her exercise program. Recently, on a TV interview, she joked about having had replacements of her knee and hip joints. I doubt that those who followed her exercise program and later needed joint replacement found it humorous. Then, there was the engineer who fancied himself a health expert and extolled believers to run after a large "carb-loading" spaghetti dinner the evening before. He died of a sudden heart attack at age fifty one, still believing that he was in perfect health. Dangerously, some runners still follow that carb-loading practice.

If it doesn't work, it doesn't work! Common sense tells us to admit that; yet, proponents of ineffective advice scold us, saying we are not trying hard enough.

Anyone can make mistakes, except big government! It rarely admits being wrong. When a corporation makes a mistake but avoids acknowledging and correcting it, it may go bankrupt. When the Federal government attempted to reduce health costs decades ago, it did so by trying to make Americans healthier. In seeking to educate us about what is healthy and what is not, it followed ineffective information, heavily twisted by industry. Today, the number of people suffering from the very conditions that the government hoped to remedy has more than doubled.

Despite this horrific failure, bureaucrats considered themselves "successful" because they did not ask the question "did disease and death increase or decrease?" to measure their success or failure. Instead, they "succeeded" since many

Chapter 3: Wrong Ideas

followed their health message. The message, although wrong, got through. That very same bureaucracy still is not open; the career bureaucrats do not admit their role in these failures. Officials in senior positions today accepted these wrong ideas when they were younger and have spent their careers defending those mistakes. Oh, about those health costs they tried to control; they doubled, too.

All of this is particularly dangerous during this new age of epidemics because many of these myths and half-truths have found their way into government policies and public beliefs. The burden of additional inflammation from chronic disease makes today's epidemic more deadly. The combination of Covid-19 inflammation and the inflammations of hidden and chronic disease can kill. You should be outraged if you are Black, Native American, or older. Even if you are not, you are not safe. Ten wrong ideas described in this chapter are those that I believe represent the greatest danger during this crisis and will continue to be dangerous on their own. Later chapters will focus on how you can change, including things to do on your own and things to do together with your physician.

Here is my list of ten wrong ideas:

1. **Most chronic disease is irreversible.**
2. **Excess *weight itself* is your true enemy.**
3. **Eat 2,000 calories each day to stay healthy.**
4. **Eating fat is bad for you.**
5. **Exercise is the best way to lose weight.**
6. **Avoiding sunlight is healthy.**

7. **Cholesterol is bad for you.**

8. **Everyone should avoid salt in their diet.**

9. **The safety of medications and food additives is well understood.**

10. **All scientific research is trustworthy.**

This chapter explains why each of these mistaken beliefs is wrong. Later chapters will focus on change that strengthens your defenses and makes you healthier.

1. Most chronic disease is irreversible.

Not true! Much chronic disease is reversible. Understanding this is essential for your Covid-19 defense. Time is crucial, so you should begin building your wall and have it in place when you need it. Often, we falsely believe that one diagnosis or another means we are doomed to forever suffer from a particular disease or condition. We think that the best we can do is tolerate a lifetime of medications, attempting to control that problem. That very belief stands in the way of taking action to change!

You must look further since there may be an underlying cause that can be modified. **Attacking the underlying cause should be your first line of defense.** It takes time and understanding for your doctor to understand you as a complex patient. It takes even more time to work, with you, to give you the teaching and guidance you may need. If your doctor has turned her back to you and focused on her computer terminal, it is not her fault. Government bureaucracy and corporate profits interfere with medical care. Her medical employer uses that computer to create the most profitable description of your

Chapter 3: Wrong Ideas

care for their insurance billing. This combination of corporate greed and an insurance nightmare dissuades doctors who really do want to take the time to listen and understand their patients' needs.

Educate your doctor. Medical care that improves your health while it reduces your need for medication produces the best possible result! Be wary of "alternative care models" if they are designed to sell you thousands of dollars of products. If possible, always keep your doctor informed and in the loop. Get your physician's attention and talk to her. Objective data can verify your success. Chapter 6 discusses objective medical tests your doctor will find helpful in understanding your improving health.

Once you succeed in making yourself healthier, stay with it. Lifestyle change means you have rapidly reversed years of a behavioral pattern. Old habits die hard, and months of your successful new behavior can easily slip away if you become too comfortable. When you are successful, acknowledge your success but remain vigilant. Be grateful for your success, but keep it up. Doing so requires a new mindset about the disease. Use the term "recovering" rather than "recovered" and consider your problems "in remission" rather than "cured." This simple change of terminology will keep you vigilant and protect you from succumbing to old temptations.

Remember, you began this book to learn how to build a protective wall against the Covid-19 epidemic. By now, you should realize you are also protecting yourself from other diseases. Treatment of one chronic disease can prevent many other medical issues, both acute and chronic. It is a continuing chain of prevention and the benefits of treatment and prevention may overlap. As an example, someone who reverses their type II diabetes greatly reduces their likelihood of heart or kidney disease. That becomes primary prevention at its best!

2. *Excess weight itself is your true enemy.*

Not exactly. The amount you weigh reflects how healthy or unhealthy you are, but it's more complex than that. For some problems, it is the cause and effect, but for others, it is concurrence. Some things, such as wearing out your joints, are a direct consequence of your weight. However, many other problems, such as diabetes, are attributed to extra weight but are really only correlated with weight.

What does that mean in plain English? Let's say you continually eat more than your body needs for energy. It would be quite natural for you to gain weight and eventually become a type II diabetic. The overweight and diabetes both seem to go together, but one did not cause the other. The two issues simply have the same underlying cause. An epidemiologist might say, "correlation does not establish causation."

That distinction matters. If you were to correct your diet in the right way, your diabetes could improve rapidly, but your weight loss could be slow and steady, taking time to lose what took years to gain. You are reversing both issues simultaneously; yet, the improvement in one is more noticeable than the other. Your health will significantly improve before you reach any magic number regarding your weight. Metabolically, you are a new person and have saved your life. People must be evaluated as individuals, their achievements recognized,

Chapter 3: Wrong Ideas

and applauded. **Healthy comes in all shapes and sizes.**

3. Eat 2,000 calories each day to stay healthy.

Nonsense. Individual needs vary, but 2,000 calories is above the energy needed for the average adult today. This is not 1940! The last time many Americans were underweight was during the Great Depression of the 1930s. When the military draft started in 1940, underweight was a major cause for rejecting new draftees. Today, overweight is a major cause of rejection for new military volunteers.

During the 1940s, the government tried to reverse that underweight problem with recommendations for a minimum daily diet. They even resorted to a campaign encouraging Americans to eat doughnuts as health food! Today's energy needs are far less than they were in 1940. High energy users of 1940, such as loggers, dock workers, and farmers, still work hard today, but mechanization has reduced their daily energy needs. More importantly, everyday tasks for the average person are vastly different. You must discover what your personal routine energy need is. Ignore those who encourage you to damage your health with outdated ideas.

4. Eating fat is bad for you.

Wrong. Fat is essential for life. Breast-fed infants generally are healthier and have a lower chance of becoming overweight or diabetic later in life. Such better health has been attributed to many things, but consider the fat content of breast milk. Although that content varies widely among individual nursing mothers, fat is the key nutrient in human breast milk.

Fat content varies from about 6% to nearly 30%! That higher percentage makes it similar to typical whipping cream. The lower percentage is closer to commercial infant formula, but still about double the percentage of fat in commercial "whole milk."

Getting enough of the right type of fat is essential for an infant's developing brain and nervous system! Certain forms of dietary fat become building blocks for your body. These are known as "essential fatty acids." In highly stratified societies, the upper classes knew the benefits of having sufficient fat in their diet, while lower classes had far less opportunity to eat fat. In the Bible, the Pharaoh of Egypt told Joseph to bring his family to Egypt, promising they would live well by stating, "they shall live off the fat of the land." Whatever your beliefs are, this illustrates a long-standing knowledge of the role of fat in eating well.

Doesn't eating fat go against the research? <u>No</u>. Research about the American diet indeed showed eating more fat coincides with health issues, but there is one serious flaw with that research. Studies done over decades (such as in Framingham, Massachusetts) looked at the amount of fat eaten by people who were typically <u>also eating a "normal" American diet containing over two pounds of sugar a week!</u> Individual sugar consumption today in America today is about twenty-five times that at the time of our nation's founding.

The presence of that high amount of sugar has caused the metabolic imbalance, leading to increased heart disease. In the presence of high sugar, more fat does increase problems, <u>but it is because of the extra sugar</u>. Very high-fat diets were

Chapter 3: Wrong Ideas

typical for native Inuit (Eskimo) populations in Alaska, northern Canada, and Greenland early in the 20th century. Lacking that high sugar intake, they were very healthy, without heart disease or diabetes. Governments "civilized" them and totally changed their diets so that their rates of diabetes are now among the highest in the world.

5. Exercise is the best way to lose weight.

No, exercise is not the best way to lose weight, but a reasonable exercise program that meets an individual's needs should be part of any weight loss program. The idea that exercise, <u>by itself,</u> is enough for most people to lose weight has been disproven by research. Yes, if you are trying to lose weight, I encourage you to exercise sensibly, but <u>in conjunction with an effective diet</u>.

People who start exercise binges to lose weight, without incorporating diet and lifestyle changes, imagine they are burning many calories. In fact, they often are burning far less than they think; yet, they reward themselves with extra food. When they do not lose weight, many simply give up. Think of all the dusty exercise machines used as clothes hangers in spare rooms and basements.

Some overweight people sometimes try to lose weight by jogging only to develop serious knee problems later in life. Sports medicine clinics, orthopedic surgeons, and physical therapists constantly see people with sports injuries paying the price for overly enthusiastic exercise programs. In some gyms, the presence of a few buff gym-goers in stylish exercise gear hurt the self-esteem of average gym-goers. Some people harm themselves, over-exercising to keep up, while others simply give up. The benefit of sane and rational exercise should belong to the average person on an average day, not just to the exceptional or pretentious few.

6. Avoiding sunlight is healthy.

No. Sunlight is essential for human life. Can it be dangerous? Yes, but avoiding it can be far more dangerous. The lack of sunlight harms millions, both physically and mentally. It confuses our immune systems, both creating inflammation and preventing appropriate response to real threats. Both of these issues might be enough to account for increased severity if infected by Covid-19.

People face very real danger when receiving high doses of ultraviolet (UV) light (from both strong natural sunlight and artificial tanning sources). Such high doses of ultraviolet light may trigger skin cancer. One type of skin cancer, melanoma, is highly dangerous and can quickly spread if not removed. Fortunately, because it is usually visible on the skin, much of the time melanoma can be removed and causes no further problems. Despite that, melanoma still kills several thousand Americans each year. If that were the entire story, avoiding total sunlight would make sense.

However, that is not the whole story. The expression "tan and healthy" came about through observation that these were often associated. Sunlight had been used medically for many purposes. A century and a half ago, patients suffering from tuberculosis were sent to locations where sunlight was abundant and kept outdoors to absorb as much as possible. Hospitals were built with a solarium, a greenhouse-like room where the patients might receive as much sunlight as possible,

Chapter 3: Wrong Ideas

even in the nastiest weather. People were treated medically with UV sunlamps, and many households regularly used them as a preventive measure. City children were sent to summer camps to get as much outdoor exposure as possible. Charities that continue to this day were initially established so that the poorest children would not be deprived of that experience.

Despite the recognition of the importance of sunlight in maintaining health, the physical mechanism was not clear. The discovery of vitamin D about a century ago changed our knowledge, but research leading to our full understanding continues to this day.[3] Today we know that Vitamin D is unlike other vitamins. It is actually a hormone, and if we are exposed to sufficient sunlight, we can make all we need. An adult with adequate sun exposure can make as many as 10,000 international units (IU) each day. The early discoveries about vitamin D focused on its role regulating calcium in the creation of strong bones. The addition of a <u>small amount</u> of vitamin D to milk was enough to prevent children from developing rickets. That is a disease where their bodies' weight kept their soft bones from growing straight and strong. That supplementation continues to this day.

In recent years we are learning that the basis for associating tanned skin with health is also due to vitamin D. Vitamin D helps regulate our immune system. Our immune system should not go crazy, injuring our tissues, nor lazy, ignoring real threats. Today, complex and mixed autoimmune disorders are common. Problems such as fibromyalgia, myositis, rheumatoid arthritis, psoriasis, and others are routine.

---

3. DeLuca, HF. **History of the discovery of vitamin D and its active metabolites.** *BoneKEy Reports* **3** Article number: 479 (2014) DOI: 10.1038/bonekey.2013.213

They are treated with powerful and often expensive drugs that disable our immune system, leaving us vulnerable when we need it to fight off genuine invaders. Our mental health is affected due to a lack of sunlight and is often associated with depression. For other functions, we need higher levels of vitamin D than that needed for strong bones.

We must use caution if taking vitamin D. It can get to be too high, something that is not a problem when we produce it within our body. During the 1930s, patent medicines were produced, having many times the normal amount of vitamin D, and some people became ill. Since then, the recommended allowance for vitamin D is set purposely low, enough to prevent calcium-related issues but too little to prevent these other problems. Fortunately, a doctor can test to see if you have the right level in your body.

Vitamin D deficiency has become a common problem in the United States and many other parts of the world. The common use of air conditioning has us spending our summer months indoors. In earlier years, homes and offices would be unbearably hot, forcing people to spend time outdoors. With air conditioning, that is no longer the case. Added to that, peoples' fear of skin cancer worsens the problem of sunlight avoidance.

7. *Cholesterol is bad for you.*

Wrong. This belief that cholesterol is bad for you has been the bedrock of "preventive" medical care for several decades but is very misguided. Only if we continue to use high levels of sugar in our diet, does lowering cholesterol help to reduce heart disease. However, the sugar industry prompted this misguided effort, which will be discussed a few pages from

Chapter 3: Wrong Ideas

now, along with issues of scientific trustworthiness. Lowering cholesterol is not nearly as effective as attacking the dietary cause of the problem. Although cholesterol is present in the plaque that may block blood vessels, it is just an ingredient and not the cause. The cause is low-level inflammation resulting from insulin resistance and metabolic syndrome. The buildup of fatty streaks and plaque is the body's attempt to heal that inflammation.

Pharmaceutical companies have produced drugs that lower total cholesterol, and by doing that, they have reinforced the idea that total cholesterol is the best indicator of cardiovascular risk. That is not true. Doctors and other scientists today know that it is the balance of cholesterol and other lipids (fatty substances in the blood) that indicate risk. Dietary change can often correct those imbalances and risk factors, but that creates no profit for influential drug manufacturers.

We also know that we can drive cholesterol too low. Low total cholesterol is associated with serious problems. Cholesterol is an important building block for many things, including adult sexual hormones. Men and women with very low cholesterol are more likely to develop depression and even commit suicide. Their sexual drive will be reduced, and women may see their menstrual cycle cease. Instead of simply seeking lower total cholesterol, learning about dietary change and working with your physician to find balance without medication is a better goal. Achieving that balance in you serum lipids can serve as a marker for reduced inflammation, and the strengthening of your protective wall.

8. All people should avoid salt in their diet.

Wrong. The average person should avoid salt <u>if their physician has instructed them to do so</u>. A legitimate reason might be congestive heart failure, kidney disease, or uncontrolled hypertension. Never put yourself on a low-salt diet because of a news article, but instead ask your doctor if you have a specific need to do so.

Four decades after the government began advising people to follow a low-salt diet, nephrologists (kidney specialists) still can not agree if this is good or bad advice for the general public. You would not take someone else's medicine just because they needed it. Why would you follow someone else's salt restriction?

A "salt" chemically contains an atom of a mineral and an atom of chlorine. Sodium, the mineral in common table salt, is essential for life and found in all our cells. The need for salt has been known for ages. Under extreme conditions of heat and heavy work, we lose minerals rapidly through sweat. At those times, we need extra minerals in our diet. In the past years, salt tablet dispensers next to water fountains were common in places where people worked or exercised vigorously. These were removed in the panic over salt, and significant problems developed. Salt tablets were quickly replaced by "sports drinks," expensive concoctions that provide similar minerals in a liquid form. We still hear of young athletes dying because they were not prepared for strenuous exercise in high heat. Keeping your minerals and your hydration adequate and balanced can keep you from becoming fatigued and confused. Allowing your hydration level and mineral

Chapter 3: Wrong Ideas

balance to be disrupted will worsen your chances, should you become ill from any cause.

What about the research? News reports often incorrectly say we put too much salt in our food. The actual studies say that we have an imbalance with too much sodium in our diet due to eating too much highly processed food! The food manufacturers adding high sodium flavor enhancers are the culprits. Reading product labels closely and understanding the chemicals in your food can make the difference (See Chapters 10-11).

There is another important additional reason to use table salt. A century ago, doctors found more people suffered from hypothyroidism in the Midwest than along either coast. People living on both coasts ate more fresh ocean fish than people in inland areas. They absorbed the mineral iodine from those fish. Their thyroid glands needed iodine to function. At first, doctors prescribed iodine solutions to those with thyroid problems but realized that iodine added to ordinary table salt would prevent this condition in many people. That worked well for decades, and iodized salt was found in every household. However, since this questionable government advice convinced many to stop using table salt, hypothyroidism is once again quite common. It is now easier for doctors to prescribe inexpensive synthetic thyroid hormone than to consider iodine relief, which is another unnatural way to ignore an underlying problem.

Strangely, this issue is well known but ignored domestically by our government. The Swiss, recognizing the problem, ordered increases in iodine in their food supply to compensate for lower iodized salt use. The World Health Organization was concerned about hypothyroidism in pregnant women, a cause of mentally disabled babies in areas of central Africa. They developed a program to distribute iodized salt to those women, and American taxes pay for much of that.

9. The safety of medications and food additives is well understood.

Sometimes we understand the safety of medications and food additives, but sometimes we do not! Safety testing of medications is built into the approval process for new drugs. However, such safety testing can never be complete. Evaluating a drug's safety for a few hundred people will only show the most obvious defects and dangers. It will not show problems that may occur only after long-term use. It will not show problems that may occur in only a few people. It will not show problems that occur when people are taking multiple drugs and they interact.

Drug trials are very expensive, so drug companies will keep them as simple as possible to obtain regulatory approval. Women and racial minorities are often underrepresented, so special issues that apply to them may not be brought to light. Sometimes, drugs later find use in children but were initially tested only in adults.

The real test of a drug begins after approval, once the drug is on the market. There is a passive reporting system so that physicians or patients may notify the Food and Drug Administration (FDA) when problems occur. Neither the physician nor the patient may be in a good position to recognize whether a problem came from a drug and report it,

Chapter 3: Wrong Ideas

so issues may take years to be recognized. Older drugs and many over-the-counter medications may have even less information available. Drugs from generic manufacturers must have the same active ingredient, but there may be slight differences. Drugs, whether manufactured in the United States or abroad, may be made from impure and untested imported chemicals, so drugs that were initially safe suddenly become dangerous and have to be recalled or taken off the market. Even everyday food, such as grapefruit, can interfere with the normal action of a drug.

The U.S. Food and Drug Administration (FDA) has no authority to evaluate so-called "nutritional supplements" unless they <u>first</u> cause serious problems. Manufacturers of such supplements are allowed to advertise the supplements as cure-alls, as long as they add a fine-print disclaimer that says they are not intended to treat or cure any disease. The situation is worse for food additives. Again, little may be known about their long-term effects. Years ago, a few food additives were highly dangerous and could cause immediate problems. The rest were considered "safe." There is a long list of items deemed "generally recognized as safe" (GRAS), which grandfathers in many items from scrutiny. Worse yet, the FDA is not the only agency involved.

Labeling for most processed foods belongs to the FDA, but meats and poultry are controlled by the Department of Agriculture (USDA) and alcoholic beverages by the Treasury Department. All three agencies have loopholes in labeling regulations allowing manufacturers to hide the real ingredients consumers might wish to avoid. Right now, knowledge is your best defense. Chapter 11 will provide you with information about labeling differences and tricks. The more you learn about labeling, the safer your choices will be.

Caveat emptor, let the buyer beware. Initial scientific reviews indicated that a few common drugs <u>might</u> partially block the Covid-19 virus from infecting cells, while other reviews indicated concern that some common drugs could worsen infection! Given this frequently changing flow of information and speculation, how can you and your physician discern what medications are both safe and useful for you?

One rule of thumb that physicians <u>used to</u> pay attention to was the more medications a person was on, the more likely adverse interactions and side effects were likely to occur. Today, as patients get older, the number of different prescription medications they take may be enormous. This is called *polypharmacy* and is made even worse when people also take herbal supplements with unknown ingredients. The best defense is to become healthier, so you need fewer and fewer medications—*caveat emptor.*

<u>10. All scientific research is trustworthy.</u>

No. It is a noble dream to believe that all scientists are equally devoted to advancing truth. Science should be a calling, attracting people who wish to spend their lives advancing knowledge and hoping to benefit humanity. That is our picture of the ideal scientist, holding multiple advanced degrees from prestigious institutions. The most revered and brilliant scientists often surpassed their education to become leaders in their field or even create new fields. Think of Benjamin Franklin, who had limited formal education; yet, he

Chapter 3: Wrong Ideas

was one of the most brilliant scientists and inventors of his day. Think of Louis Pasteur, who was trained as a chemist, then became a pioneer in the new field of microbiology and a developer of medical treatment. At the other end of the spectrum, we have always had those scientists whose desire for self-aggrandizement, money, and position were more important than advancing truth and benefiting humanity.

As an example, many of the negative consequences of tobacco use were known in the 1600s. Still, until the 1990s, that did not stop tobacco companies from finding scientists who would say tobacco did no harm in return for generous compensation. The tobacco giants used these "scientists" to delay being held responsible for generations.

More recently, early in the Covid-19 pandemic, there was interest in using inexpensive generic drugs that some thought might be useful as protection against serious infection. There was also interest in very expensive new antiviral drugs, potentially worth billions in profits to pharmaceutical companies. The World Health Organization (WHO) began to conduct an international cooperative trial to see if one particular inexpensive drug was of any use. Suddenly, papers were published by two of the most respected medical journals in the world. These papers claimed that the inexpensive drug was ineffective and dangerous. Supposedly, this was based upon the medical records of tens of thousands of patients. A team of scientists supposedly reviewed those records. Two of those scientists were at prestigious institutions, and one had been the recipient of many contracts and grants involving drug companies. The third scientist worked for a company that supposedly had a huge database with worldwide inpatient hospital records. Based upon this, many hospitals and doctors quickly stopped trying the cheap drug and focused on experimenting with the newer expensive medicines. The FDA withdrew its stamp of approval for evaluating the cheap drug to be tried for Covid-19. WHO called off its effort to try to determine if that older drug was useful. It seemed to many, particularly political pundits and news outlets, that the question had been answered.

Those who read the studies were confused. If true, it was important information, but there were some puzzling and unanswered questions about the data itself. No one seemed to know that this large database had even existed before these papers appeared! Hospitals where patients were supposedly treated had no idea how data from their institution could have ended up in this reported database. As people questioned and investigated, problems became obvious. Once questions were voiced, even the co-authors denied responsibility for their own study, claiming that they had not actually seen the data; they had simply relied upon summaries provided by the third author, the one who was affiliated with the company holding the supposed information. In truth, it quickly became apparent that all the data was fictitious. The supposed data existed in only in the imagination of one scientist. The prestigious medical journals quickly retracted the published articles. Because genuine research was called off, it delayed answering an important question about how people should be treated at a critical time.

Could there have been hidden reasons, such as

shutting down research into a rival product? At this time, we still don't know the reasons for this fictitious science and we may never learn them. **What we do know is that two of the most prestigious peer-reviewed medical journals in the world got taken in.** If that can happen to them, how can the average person spot a fake!

Another important fake concerns diet. During the late 1970s, the government began promoting certain dietary changes that have proven to be disastrous, whether they admit it or not. They thought they were doing the right thing, relying on what they considered a body of evidence claiming that fat was unhealthy. It was bogus, and it contradicted thousands of years of knowledge in both medicine and agriculture. Yet, the prestige of this "new scientific data" swayed the government. Not until 2016[4] was it revealed that the sugar industry had lucrative contracts with leading nutritional scientists. In exchange for money, the sugar industry could censor and block publication of studies showing excess sugar consumption was the villain. Instead, they could encourage pointing the finger unfairly at dietary fat. The epidemic of excess weight and type II diabetes that resulted has led to suffering and death. It appears this did not happen by accident.

That being said, whom should you trust? **It is important not to be swayed by information that contradicts what you can see happening with your own eyes.**

---

4. Glantz S et al. **Sugar Industry and Coronary Heart Disease Research A Historical Analysis of Internal Industry Documents** . *JAMA Intern Med.* 2016;176 (11):1680-1685. doi:10.1001/jamainternmed.2016.5394

Chapter 4

The Inflammatory Spectrum of Diabetes.

"I saw few die of hunger; of eating 100,000."
Benjamin Franklin
in the voice of *Poor Richard*, 1736

Many chronic problems that cause inflammation fall on a timeline that gradually leads to type II diabetes. This spectrum of problems has received many names over the years as if each were a separate entity. Over the ages, the terminology has changed. Some of these names attempt to describe a complete picture while others are the results of the complex development of type II diabetes: λειουρία (leiouría), prameha, zuckerkranken, adult-onset diabetes, insulin resistance, metabolic syndrome, polycystic ovary syndrome, hyperglycemia, syndrome X, the deadly quartet, the insulin-resistance syndrome, and peripheral neuropathy.

You may have heard of some of these, and others may be new to you. You might have thought that some of these were separate entities, but they are all related, points along the same line, parts of the wide spectrum of diabetes. If a test ordered by your doctor did not reach the threshold for the

Chapter 4: The Inflammatory Spectrum of Diabetes

"official" diagnosis of diabetes, you might have been told everything was normal, and you felt safe. Unless the correct tests were ordered and properly interpreted, nothing could be further from the truth.

Long before type II diabetes is diagnosed, its spectrum of complications is harmful. Add the inflammation of Covid-19 to this inflammation, and you have a recipe for disaster. These are not just a prelude to danger. These are a real danger. The mistake we make is considering these separate entities and not recognizing them as points on a lethal timeline.

Understanding the difference between type I and type II diabetes is important. Despite sounding alike, they describe vastly different problems. You may have heard about Doctors Banting and Best, Canadian physicians who discovered insulin in 1924. They experimented with a dog, removed its pancreas and created a diabetic dog. The dog could not process the sugar in its diet, and its blood-sugar level went up. Later, they injected the ground-up pancreas into the dog, and its sugar level fell. They showed that a substance in the dog's pancreas was capable of lowering blood sugar.

That substance was insulin, which came from the insulin producing beta cells of the pancreas. The experiment of Drs. Banting and Best mimicked type I diabetes. Type I diabetes is a catastrophic event. The body simply stops producing sufficient insulin due to an attack damaging to the pancreas or its control mechanism. Injecting insulin will lower blood sugar in anyone, whether they are healthy, a type I diabetic, or a type II diabetic. Even though today only about 5 percent of all people with diabetes are type I diabetics, many people still think of all forms of diabetes as a disease of insulin insufficiency.

Type II diabetes is vastly different. In some ways, it is the exact opposite of type I diabetes. Type II diabetes is a progressive disease with a gradual, insidious onset. Insulin insufficiency, if it occurs at all, occurs later in the course of the disease and is not total but relative to the needs of the individual. I prefer to use the term "**diabetic spectrum disorder.**" That name describes all the things that are happening long before the traditional diagnosis of diabetes. Damage is occurring all along that timeline.

Objective tests can demonstrate this early damage if they are used. Many routine diabetes tests miss this completely. Chapter 6 will provide information about tests that will help you and your doctor. Government health authorities are just beginning to pay attention to some of the earlier stages of diabetes, but in the wrong way. You may have heard the term "prediabetes" being used recently. That very name "pre-diabetes" trivializes the danger. People who are told they have pre-diabetes may mistakenly understand it to warn of a future event. They may not realize the harm it is causing right now. I ask women who were told they were pre-diabetic whether, during their first trimester of pregnancy, their physician called them "pre-pregnant?" That may bring a laugh, but then, they get it.

Since ancient times, people have recognized diabetes as a disease. Diabetes or *prameha* (an ancient Sanskrit word) describes excessive urinary flow. One form of diabetes, *diabetes mellitus*, describes urine that is also sweet. Physicians

Chapter 4: The Inflammatory Spectrum of Diabetes

saw flies attracted to that urine of patients and discovered it was sweet. Not until the 19th century did it become clear that people already had high sugar levels in their blood before it "spilled" into their urine. Since then, we have used the blood sugar (glucose) level above a certain point as the definition of diabetes. With type II diabetes, that definition ignores all the bad things that occur long before reaching that point.

The progression of type II diabetes follows a logical sequence. First, a person may eat more than their body immediately needs. As their blood sugar level rises, their pancreas quickly responds by creating more insulin in its beta cells and sends it off through their bloodstream. That insulin has several important roles. When cells need energy (in the form of glucose), the insulin allows the cells to take it up and use it.

Another purpose of insulin is to signal to your liver that you have excess energy. Your liver is your body's major chemical factory. Compare it to an industrial refinery. A refinery takes in raw petroleum and converts it to many forms, such as gasoline, jet fuel, diesel oil, and industrial petrochemicals. Similarly, your liver constantly manipulates and changes the form of energy that your body takes in.

When you overeat and have too much energy in your diet, a small amount is converted into ready, short-term energy. That short-term reserve is a starch called *glycogen*. Glycogen can instantly be turned back into glucose for a quick rise in blood sugar, which is very useful for emergency energy. Larger amounts of extra energy get turned into fat. Fat is an important long-term energy element because it is an efficient and compact way to store a lot of energy until it is needed. Your body tries to keep fat for periods of starvation, so it favors burning sugar when that is plentiful. That is how animals prepare for the winter, taking in extra energy and building up their body fat to be used when food is scarce.

Humans have the same mechanism and used it regularly in more primitive agricultural times. Such fat was often needed since winter scarcity could mean you would starve without enough stored fat. Most of us in industrialized nations live in a different world today. Mass-scale agriculture, transportation, food preservation, and distribution all negate the need for a large fat supply to get through the winter! Our bodies rarely need to turn to that mass of stored energy. Even the chemical pathways that allow us to use fat become inefficient from lack of use efficiently.

The fat your liver produces is called a *triglyceride*, and as it produces it, the same insulin signal also tells your body to send fat into storage. All of those extra triglycerides being created and moved around temporarily will show up in a blood test. So far, everything described is perfectly normal. Your body produced extra insulin when needed to get the job done, but it was a temporary event. No harm, no foul!

But what if this were not a single event? What if overeating was routine and your body frequently produced more insulin to control that extra unneeded energy? Imagine that you worked for an abusive supervisor. How would you feel when your boss shouted at you? The first time, you might jump and pay attention! What if that behavior happened routinely? Would you adapt to it? Would you be irritated and start to tune

Chapter 4: The Inflammatory Spectrum of Diabetes

out your boss? Now, use this analogy to picture what happens to your cells when they are constantly bombarded with high insulin levels. They begin to tune out the message of insulin. They lose sensitivity to it. We call this **insulin resistance**.

Insulin resistance is the beginning of trouble. If your cells get tired of hearing the same message from insulin repeatedly, they work less efficiently. They don't do as much work as they should. That reduction in responsiveness would keep your sugar level too high, except that your pancreas adjusts and works even harder, creating even more insulin. It would be like your supervisor shouting even louder to get you moving. At first, this works within your body. Your blood sugar does not seem to go very high. If we use a test for your average blood sugar, it may still seem okay. In contrast, if we tested for the amount of insulin that was needed to keep that blood sugar normal, that test would show that your insulin level was abnormally high.

This excess production of insulin by your own body is how type II diabetes starts. This makes type II diabetes very different than type I diabetes. In type I diabetes, from the very beginning, you had insufficient insulin and your sugar level was high. Type II diabetes is just the opposite. Your blood sugar may still be normal at this early stage, but your insulin level is high.

Although this is an early stage, it can easily be a killer. As part of the *metabolic syndrome*, insulin resistance creates inflammation. Inflammation occurs in your blood vessels. That inflammation causes fatty streaks in vessels as your body tries to heal that inflammation. Eventually, those could turn into plaque and interfere with the blood flow to your organs. Abnormal amounts of chemicals called *cytokines* would be produced. Cytokines are signaling proteins that tell our immune system how to react, controlling inflammation and immune response to infection. Finding abnormal levels of triglycerides, fat produced by our liver, circulating in our blood is a marker for this imbalance, as is an excess of a protein called C-reactive protein (CRP).

Despite all this, you likely would feel "normal" and not know that these changes were occurring. You might have said to yourself, "I am just putting on a little weight as I mature, but it happens to everyone in my family." Just noticing the fat being deposited around your body should be enough reason to look further. Chapter 6 will explain how you can have objective proof if any abnormality exists by being tested for the right markers in your blood.

A high insulin level makes your body store extra fat in your mid-section, which we call *central obesity*. Extra fat is attached to an apron-like organ called your *omentum*, a Latin word for apron. This deep omental fat covers your abdominal organs and changes your shape. Compare this to an apple's shape, bulging in the middle, rather than a pear, which is plumper at the bottom. American men with waistlines over 40 inches and women with waistlines over 36 inches are considered to have this problem. If your ancestry is Asian, Native American, or Latin American, your safe numbers are even lower. Men, this means your actual waist size, not the size of pants you purchase to wear well below your belly.

At this stage, **"learned helplessness"** often rears its

Chapter 4: The Inflammatory Spectrum of Diabetes

ugly head. When people begin to gain weight and cannot do anything about it, many blame themselves. Earlier, I said that healthy comes in many shapes and sizes. The same can be said for physical beauty or attractiveness. In our society, this hurts women earlier than it does men. Notions of what is ideal have varied across cultures and periods. Just compare the curvy models in the 17th-century paintings by Reubens to the anorexic-looking model Twiggy of the 1960s.

When a weight gain seems impossible to control, people may blame themselves, but they often are victims of both food addiction and the food-processing industry. One unfortunate mental defense that these victims may turn to is the proposition that not being able to control their weight is normal. It is *not* normal, and believing that it is okay is dangerous for your health.

You can fight back. What you need is the correct knowledge of the steps you must take. If, instead, you allow the false knowledge that created the problem in the first place to guide you, you cannot win. The frustration and self-blame from sticking to old ideas become barriers to getting healthy. To understand this, let's talk about addiction. Addiction is a loaded word, bringing with it visions of heroin addicts and needles. I am going to presume that no one ever grew up saying, "I plan to be overweight when I become an adult." Actually, no heroin addicts who I ever met said that they dreamed of drug addiction as their future when they were young either!

Let's start by defining some terms. Hunger and starvation are vastly different words, which are frequently misused. Starvation means you are not getting enough nutrients to survive. Hunger, on the other hand, means that your body is telling you to eat more. Dramatic statistics that imply a certain percentage of the population is hungry can represent starvation in less-developed nations during a famine. Starvation is still possible but less likely in developed nations with nutritional safety nets. Many people counted as "hungry" in those circumstances are not actually starving. Instead, they are suffering from a false signal telling them to eat more. If you are overweight and hungry, you are not starving. Your body has an ample energy reserve but is not using it.

How does hunger control you and cause you to gain weight? Your insulin production is an important factor. A frequent complaint from people who have to take insulin injections is that they find themselves gaining weight. Insulin has a complex variety of roles. Importantly, it makes your blood sugar level come down. Certain foods have a "high glycemic index," meaning they make your sugar level shoot up rapidly. As you eat such food, your body sends lots of insulin into your blood rapidly. That brings your sugar level down, sometimes too quickly. If your brain runs on sugar, rapidly dropping sugar levels provoke hunger, which is *reactive hypoglycemia*.

That level does not have to get extremely low, as in true hypoglycemia or low blood sugar. Instead, it is the sudden drop that triggers a reaction telling you to eat more. You may have mild anxiety and focus on food. This is a normal mechanism, reminding you to do something, but can be an overreaction when you are eating foods that cause rapid swings in your blood sugar levels. For example, if you have a high carbohydrate breakfast in the morning, such as sugar-

Chapter 4: The Inflammatory Spectrum of Diabetes

sweetened cereal or jam-covered toast, you might find yourself hungry by midmorning. If you skip breakfast entirely, you might not be able to focus on your job or schoolwork until your morning snack.

Once you have that snack, you get a quick shot of rising blood sugar and feel better, more alert, and calmer. This is a physical event, but it can easily cross over into a psychological addiction as well. When that sugar-laden treat makes you feel better, you remember that reaction. This type of eating pattern easily becomes addictive. You may search for that good feeling other times you are feeling upset. Turning to food when you are upset becomes a pattern. Satisfaction from such an emotion-laden food craving may lead you to falsely think you can not get along without some particular treat.

Recent changes in agriculture, transportation, and food chemistry have all created a greater likelihood of getting hooked on food. Some food companies are reported to employ brain chemistry experts to make food more addictive. These may be the same folks that were or are employed by big tobacco companies to make their product more addictive.[5] Food's ability to become addictive is not new but is much more common today than in ancient times.

When certain foods were affordable only by the rich and powerful, the epidemics of obesity and diabetes that these brought stood out more in those groups. Today, this form of cheap and plentiful danger is available throughout society.

---

5. Callahan P, et al. **Where there's smoke, there might be food research, too,** *Chicago Tribune*, January 29, 2006.
www.chicagotribune.com/bussiness/chi-0601290254jan29,0,1306987.story (accessed 30 Jan 2007)

Fighting Covid-19, the Unequal Opportunity Killer

Those who are poorer have more than their share! Insulin resistance is common when your diet relies heavily on traditionally abundant and cheap carbohydrate-laden foods. If you already have insulin resistance, once you become infected with the Covid-19 virus, it will cause you greater harm and danger.

Moving on to the next phase of this disorder, as your insulin resistance worsens, your pancreas struggles to keep up with insulin production. If it takes longer to produce enough insulin to pull your sugar level back; your average sugar level will go up. That is easily detectable using the right blood test, hemoglobin A1c, which will be explained in chapter 6. Even though your average sugar level is too high, your sugar may still return to normal after many hours, so your morning sugar level will seem low enough. If doctors only test your fasting glucose, without checking your A1c, they will miss the problem. Instead, they might wrongly reassure you that you do not have diabetes.

Eventually, you may reach the stage where your body can no longer keep your sugar level down after an overnight fast. Finally, an abnormality will be detected, and you will be called *diabetic*. The truth is, you may have been somewhere on the spectrum of diabetes for years.

That is the reason I use the term **diabetic spectrum disorder.** Long before a diabetes diagnosis is reached, the "low-grade inflammation" related to insulin resistance was present. That inflammation raises your risk of a serious and potentially deadly course if you become infected with COVID-19. It also can account for many conditions you could develop;

yet, the underlying problem may be undiagnosed or ignored. You could have developed polycystic ovary disorder with excessive acne, troublesome facial hair, and menstrual difficulties. Or perhaps, you may have found yourself infertile. You may have developed peripheral neuropathy with a loss of feeling or pain in your feet and legs. You may have developed heart or kidney disease. All these are good reasons to say that you were still on the path to becoming diabetic but were already suffering from its complications and consequences. You simply had not reached the ancient definition of flies landing in your sweet urine!

You need to understand that anywhere along this timeline, low-grade inflammation is harming you. Anywhere along this timeline, an infection from the Covid-19 virus can piggyback on an existing problem and turn deadly. Reversing this and other sources of inflammation protect you in two ways. You will be protected from the future diagnosis of type II diabetes and its associated problems. At the same time, you have toughened yourself, moving further from the high-risk group if you do become infected with Covid-19.

Chapter 5

Evaluating Your Status

You are best-qualified to consider if you are having a problem since you know things about yourself that others do not. Once you do your evaluation, your physician might have the ability to interpret what you have found. This chapter will help you look at yourself and identify reasons you should get your physician to order certain objective laboratory tests. Inflammation from insulin resistance and low vitamin D leading to a dysfunctional immune system are two problems that can be identified with lab testing. If detected, you can correct these problems yourself and strengthen your defense against Covid-19. Doing so will also protect you from many other chronic health problems and help improve some problems you already have. All you have to do now is ask yourself questions that signal whether you might need a few laboratory tests. Even if you cannot get testing done readily, these questions will make you aware of whether you should consider further action.

The first question is, *"What is your weight?"* Asking about your weight seems routine, but your weight alone is only a starting point. Often weight and "BMI" are the only criteria that a doctor's office will use. BMI stands for Body Mass Index,

Chapter 5: Evaluating Your Status

and people are judged and labeled overweight or obese due to their BMI.

BMI was invented about two centuries ago as a measure of health. It simply provides a range of purportedly ideal weights for people of a certain height. It is a statistical tool that never should have been used for individual recommendations. For over a century, physicians had a much better way to judge whether a person's weight was ideal. Life insurance companies had developed real data that actuarially estimated health. Their accumulated statistical data was based on experience with hundreds of thousands of people over many decades. Those insurers issued detailed tables, frequently used by doctors.

BMI use today is an unfortunate result of the limitations of computer technology half a century ago. Those tables were too detailed for the size of most computers at that time. Governments and scientists were anxious to use computers and began to use the antiquated BMI formula since it only involved a simple equation that could fit the smallest computer. Since this lazy use of BMI became standardized worldwide, many doctors today may no longer realize that better options for judging individual people exist and could be used.

BMI should be limited to those epidemiologists and statisticians who analyze large groups. It is a weak tool for your individual health evaluation and planning. The reason is simple. The old insurance tables had separate data, characterized by sex, age, ethnicity, and physical fitness. These distinctions do not even exist within the BMI. For example, a twenty-year-old female computer programmer of Thai ancestry would be

Fighting Covid-19, the Unequal Opportunity Killer

evaluated by BMI on the same scale as a forty-year-old male logger of Scandinavian ancestry. At best, use BMI only as a starting point.

Remember, too, weight alone is only an <u>indirect</u> measure of health. The relationship between weight and health shows correlation but not causation. As an example, let's say I have two patients. The first, who I see for the first time, is 5'10" tall and weighs 230 pounds. Using his height and weight, his BMI would classify him as obese and at high risk regarding his health. Laboratory tests might confirm his high risk.

In contrast, a second patient is a man of the same age, height, and weight as the first. The difference is that this is not the first visit for him. A year earlier, he weighed 300 pounds. Since then, he has followed a dietary plan that changed his metabolism and allowed him to lose weight. Doing the same laboratory testing on this second man would show that <u>today</u> he is at lower than average risk for disease, and his markers indicating chronic inflammation are all normal.

Nevertheless, when you visit your doctor, weight and BMI will be used to label you. If you have been told your BMI, remember it. If not, you can get it with an online "BMI calculator." The actual formula (using U.S. measurements) is your weight in pounds times 703 divided by your height in inches squared.

However you obtain it, if your BMI is between 18.5 and 24.9, you are called *normal;* between 25 and 29.9, you are labeled *overweight,* and if 30 or above, you will be portrayed as *obese.* BMI and weight should only be starting points, although they might offer the first hint that your metabolism has created

Chapter 5: Evaluating Your Status

a risk of your health being harmed from inflammation.

Waist measurement is a more specific indicator of your risk than weight. A high insulin level resulting from insulin resistance creates central obesity. It causes deep omental fat (also called visceral fat) to cover your abdominal organs and changes your shape. American men with waistlines more than 40 inches and women with waistlines over 35 inches have central obesity. If your ancestry is Asian or Latin American, those limits drop to 35½ for a man and 31½ for a woman. You can easily measure this at home, or your doctor's office can check this. Measure your actual waist size, not the clothing size of low-slung pants.

Some physicians compare a person's shape to either an apple, bulging in the middle of a pear, which is a plumper at the bottom. If your waist is wider than your hips, this too can mean higher risk.

Another measure, estimating what percentage of your body weight comes from fat, can warn you of high risk. This measure is especially useful if you want to set a weight-loss goal that is both realistic and healthy. However, there are several methods of measuring, and some of the most common methods have weaknesses. One method that was once considered the most accurate is "hydrostatic weighing." Do not try this at home! By comparing your weight normally and again completely submerged underwater, it is possible to tell how much of your body consists of fat. However, since your lungs contain air, unless the measurement is coupled with a measurement of your lung capacity, it can be inaccurate and misleading.

Fighting Covid-19, the Unequal Opportunity Killer

A method common in research involves using radiologic scans of various types, including X-Ray, CT, MRI, and DEXA. Although considered accurate, it is a research tool. It is expensive, and there is no justification for exposing yourself to unnecessary radiation to obtain this information.

The quickest and simplest method used in gymnasiums and doctor's' offices for years is the skin caliper. Your skin is pinched, and the thickness is measured at several points. Calculations then provide the percentage of fat in your body, which is a common method but is limited to only the type of fat directly under your skin, your "subcutaneous fat." It does not measure the most important health indicator, deep omental body fat, which would alert you to dangerous insulin resistance.

A newer method measures fat by sending small currents of varying frequency between your hands and your feet. A small computer chip within a scale combines that with information about your height, weight, age, and sex to calculate the percentage of your weight from fat, with a separate estimate of deep omental fat. Avoid cheaper models of electronic scales, which can only measure your lower body fat sending currents from one foot to the other. Accurate models that measure both your upper and lower body may be available at a gym, a doctor's office, and on more expensive home scales.

As a double-check, you might compare an electronic scale measurement with a caliper measurement. The difference between the total fat from these two separate measurements can also provide you another approximation of your deep omental fat. Think of the difference between the

Chapter 5: Evaluating Your Status

apple and the pear. It is the central obesity from deep omental fat that is most associated with inflammation and health risk.

Whether it is BMI, weight, percentage body fat, waist measurement, or omental fat percentage, <u>any</u> of these should be a red flag to get the appropriate blood tests for insulin resistance. In addition to these physical issues, consider your family's medical history. Do you have relatives with type II diabetes? Do you have relatives who developed heart disease at a young age? What about your health history? Have you had hypoglycemic episodes? Has your doctor ever said anything to you about diabetes, whether it was prediabetes, borderline diabetes, or gestational diabetes? Have you had heart problems, kidney problems, or peripheral neuropathy? Women, have you had ovarian problems, infertility, menstrual problems, excessive acne, or facial hair? Any of these can also be a marker for insulin resistance and a reason to be tested.

See your physician to obtain the objective blood tests, which are explained in the next chapter. Getting testing done will give you an objective measure of your issues. It will also provide a baseline to compare and to evaluate progress as your health improves. As you reduce insulin resistance and its inflammation, you lessen the damage that would occur should infection strike. However, if you can't get a test done promptly, you should still proceed with the lifestyle changes that you will be guided through in this book.

The next item to consider should be your vitamin D status. The bad news is that many people in the United States are deficient in vitamin D and are not aware of it. Vitamin D deficiency can cause significant problems with your immune system by not protecting you when it is supposed to and by over-protecting you by attacking your healthy tissues. The good news is that this can be corrected very easily. Here are some hints that you may be low. Any of these gives you a reason to be tested. This list is long, and a yes answer to any of these questions is enough to suggest you get tested.

Do you live North of the so-called Sun Belt states or 33° latitude? Over time, human skin color and our chemical systems for generating vitamin D developed to match the part of the world our ancestors came from. Experts claim that Americans living above 33° latitude do not get enough sunlight. The reason for that is due to the angle sunlight hits the earth at more northern locations. Sunlight hitting the earth at an angle has to travel through more atmosphere, limiting the amount of ultraviolet radiation reaching our skin. In the United States, 33° latitude is a line extending roughly from Southern Georgia through Northern Texas to Southern California. Even here, differences in weather can be limiting factors, as can altitude, so there is really no magic locator that guarantees enough sunlight.

Do you live in an air-conditioned home? Do you prefer to stay indoors during the summer? Do you avoid going outdoors in the middle of the day? Decades ago, when I was a younger person, air conditioning was a luxury. In the summertime heat, houses would become unbearably hot. Some people would resort to sleeping on their outdoor fire escapes or their flat roofs in large cities. (That is an ancient practice, since the Bible in Deuteronomy 22:8 warns people to build a parapet on their roof so that people will not accidentally

Chapter 5: Evaluating Your Status

roll off!) It was common for people to find reasons to be outdoors during the day, which was usually cooler. Today, people have become accustomed to air-conditioned homes and businesses, so they spend much less time outdoors. Summer is when people should be building up a stored reserve of vitamin D. Even when people go outside; many avoid the strong midday sun. Here again, the experts have something to say. The time from about 10 AM to 3 PM (using actual geographic "Sun Time" for your location) is when the sun's angle allows more passage of ultraviolet light needed for natural vitamin D generation.

Do you use sunscreen? If you do, you are trying to do the right thing. What you may not know is that you are caught between two groups of experts. On the one hand, dermatologic oncologists whose focus is cancer concentrate on sunlight and ultraviolet avoidance. The message that is picked by the press and government is that less sun exposure is always better. In contrast, dermatologic endocrinologists, who are **experts on the complex biochemistry of the skin itself**[6] **urge moderation and sensible sunlight exposure**. They recommend that people limit daily sun exposure to half the time that could cause mild sunburn. It is excessive exposure that is likely to damage the DNA and RNA within your skin. That damage can lead to premature skin aging and even cancer. These experts also point out that in addition to generating vitamin D, moderate exposure helps a system that seems to heal DNA breaks! They then say that once you reach this exposure limit, it is wise to use sunscreen for the rest of that

---

6. For a complete discussion of this complex issue, see: Wacker M, Holick M. **Sunlight and Vitamin D, A global perspective for health.** *Dermato-Endocrinology,* 2013 Jan 1; 5(1): 51-108. doi: 10.4161/derm.24494

day. Their warning does make sense, since it is impossible to determine a set amount of time that could work for everyone in our genetically diverse nation. Caution and compromise are called for in this debate. Fortunately, by monitoring your vitamin D status, you can determine your need for a supplement to make up for a Vitamin D deficiency.

What shade is your skin? Melanin pigment in your skin can filter ultraviolet light, so the same sun exposure will provide vastly different results in different people. Genetic heritage does matter here, but science unfortunately confuses racial labels based upon historic prejudices with reality. Limiting yourself to half of what might give you a sunburn is a suggestion from experts that makes more sense than using racial labels that fail to describe you.

Are you diabetic? Are you overweight? If you answered yes to either or both of these, you have a statistically higher chance of also being low in vitamin D. If you answered yes to the hints in the earlier section about insulin resistance, you probably belong here too. Checking your vitamin D level is wise.

Do you have any known autoimmune disorder such as rheumatoid arthritis, psoriasis, lupus, multiple sclerosis, myositis, fibromyalgia, or any other possibly autoimmune issue? Autoimmune diseases all represent complicated breakdowns by a confused immune system. Normally, your immune system is vigilant in protecting you from foreign invaders and defective entities in your own body. When the control system goes awry, instead of defending you, it attacks your healthy cells. Vitamin D is an important part of the control

Chapter 5: Evaluating Your Status

mechanism for your immune system. When Vitamin D is extremely low, strange things happen. It is similar to your erratically acting computer when electrical power is very low.

Rheumatologists are experts who frequently deal with these disorders. They use groups of laboratory tests to distinguish one autoimmune disease from another. Despite that, they may run into situations where the pattern of abnormal lab tests does not follow the textbook. Instead, your immune system acts as if it has its circuits crossed! Some autoimmune disorders seem more common today than decades ago when low vitamin D was less common.

With a newer disorder, such as fibromyalgia, patients were sent to psychiatrists at first because experts could not identify a physical cause. They were told they suffered from a mental problem! If you have or suspect you have had any autoimmune issue and your vitamin D level has not already been investigated, get it checked as soon as you can.

Do you have a history of cancer, tuberculosis, or heart disease? Statistically, there is a relationship. If you have suffered from any of these, please get your vitamin D level checked. The mechanisms differ, and we still do not know all we need to know about how and why. In the case of certain cancers, it is believed that in the early stages, when your immune system could have stopped a small aberration from becoming actual cancer, it did not do its job. Certain infectious diseases such as tuberculosis and other mycobacteria are often common in some third-world countries, yet the disease is not always aggressive. It seems that people's immune systems can hold the mycobacteria in check for long periods. That is the reason we screen seemingly healthy immigrants from those countries, looking for latent tuberculosis.

Vitamin D deficiency seems to allow latent tuberculosis to break free and cause disease. A century and a half ago, when tuberculosis patients at sanitariums were forced to sit outside in sunlight, no matter the weather, doctors might not have understood the mechanism of the disease, but they did recognize its pattern. This is important today when there are strains of tuberculosis resistant to most of the anti-tuberculosis drugs that science has invented.

Have you had any mental health issues, particularly depression? Here too, scientists see a pattern or believe there is a relationship between low Vitamin D and depression and strive to find the underlying causes. If you have had any mental health issues, it will not hurt to have your vitamin D level checked again.

Many people will answer yes to one of these questions. If so, get the vitamin D test done. That test is explained in the next chapter. Find out if you need extra Vitamin D. If you have a deficiency, there is an easy fix. Vitamin D is such an important messenger for your immune system that a low vitamin D level could cause severe illness if you become infected by Covid-19. In addition to the danger of Covid-19, a hidden vitamin D deficiency could be an underlying factor in many other serious problems.

In this chapter, we discussed reasons to be suspicious and to get tested for two serious and common problems, insulin resistance and low vitamin D. There are other things you can look at. Still, these are so important to your health that I will not

Chapter 5: Evaluating Your Status

waste your time with smaller issues. If you can improve in both of these areas, expect to benefit in three ways.

First, you will have hardened yourself so that if Covid-19 infects you, you will have a better chance of having a mild case.

Next, you will be doing a lot to prevent many other chronic diseases in the future.

Finally, you may find that certain chronic diseases you already have are improving.

Don't hesitate. Work with your physician to get tested, as recommended in the next chapter. Any abnormalities discovered give you solid and objective data. In the future you can compare these results to follow-up tests after you have changed your lifestyle. That objective data will demonstrate that you are doing the right things for yourself and keep the skeptics and scoffers at bay. As you become healthier, use that as hard proof so you will get the recognition you deserve. If you find that you are not able to get tested promptly, you can still safely move on and take action that will improve your health and strengthen your defenses.

Chapter 6

Objective Testing

In the last chapter, you considered whether to ask your doctor for objective testing. If you have insurance coverage[7] the last chapter should have given you valid reasons to be tested. Use those reasons to explain to your doctor why you believe these are important.

If you believe you may be **at risk for insulin resistance** or any other abnormality in the broad spectrum of type II diabetes, the following five tests should be done together. These are "first thing in the morning fasting tests":

1. **Fasting Insulin level**
2. **Comprehensive Metabolic Chemistry Panel**
3. **High Sensitivity C-Reactive Protein**
4. **Hemoglobin-A1c**
5. **Lipid Profile**

---

7. Do not go outside of your insurance coverage to get tested without checking the cost. Laboratory charges without insurance coverage in the United States can be overwhelming. You may find yourself facing a bill of hundreds of dollars if you do not use insurance coverage. Having the same tests initiated by your doctor through insurance might only cost a few dollars for a co-payment. The reasons for this are complex and have to do with the insurance companies' and the government's payment model.

Chapter 6:   Objective Testing

If you feel you may have **a low vitamin D level**, have your physician also request these next two tests. If these are the only tests done, you will not need to fast:

6. Vitamin D Level (25-Hydroxy)

7. Erythrocyte Sedimentation Rate

Your doctor might choose to do additional tests, but don't skip the important ones given here. If time allows, your doctor might also review your own and your family's medical history and do a thorough physical examination.

This chapter explains what these recommended tests are and why they are important to you. Don't forget to obtain access to or get copies of your actual results for your records. Do not accept a simple summary that only says your results were "good" or "bad." Actual results provide you objective information and are a starting point for comparing future changes and progress.

Interpreting that information is important. A report may show a numeric value and show a supposed "normal range" of values. The definition of "normal" may vary considerably, and some tests must be interpreted differently for specific conditions.

Newer research might suggest test interpretations not yet included in the typical laboratory report. Your doctor might compare a test result to an earlier test, where the direction or trend of the test might be very important, whether or not within the normal range. Sometimes, "normal" is only a statistical term showing where your results fall compared to everyone else's larger population. When the population has a high percentage of people who are developing a problem, their test results create a "population curve" that is actually "skewed" or lopsided. A skewed curve is similar to a teacher mistakenly grading on a curve when a class is actually composed of mostly very bright and hard-working students. Calling someone either normal or abnormal by comparing them to such skewed results is wrong, and doing so may miss identifying people who could be helped. The best answer is for you to review the test result to see how that information might help you.

1. Your Fasting Insulin Level. Chapter 3 discussed why many people falsely believe that diabetes means that you simply lack enough insulin. For the 95 percent of known diabetics in the United States that are type II diabetics, it is far more complex.

Type II diabetes is initially characterized by insulin resistance. Your body reacts to a high sugar level by forcing your pancreas to produce **extra insulin**. The cells that receive that high insulin signal gradually become more resistant to that insulin excess. As your insulin resistance increases, your pancreas has to produce even greater amounts of insulin to cope. That high insulin level is measurable and objective.

That cycle worsens until the later stages of type II diabetes. Eventually, your pancreas cannot produce enough insulin to keep up with the higher need caused by insulin resistance. That is the time when your increasing sugar level might come to the attention of doctors. That is also when you begin to meet the official definition of diabetes or prediabetes.

A high fasting insulin level can objectively show

Chapter 6: Objective Testing

that you have insulin resistance in the earliest stages of the diabetic spectrum, long before diagnosing prediabetes or type II diabetes.

Since you are concerned about hardening your body by reducing pre-existing inflammation, insulin resistance should be at the top of your warning list. Whether you are protecting yourself from Covid-19 or other chronic diseases, inflammation can be the real killer. With Covid-19, when the hyper-inflammation it causes is added to any pre-existing inflammation, it can prove deadly. With other chronic diseases, inflammation can be the silent killer, gradually causing deterioration of your heart, kidneys, and other organs before you recognize a problem.

The actual number you see on your laboratory report is most important since the "normal range" shown for many tests may be wrong, because it is based upon a skewed population, where so many people are ticking time bombs. Objective research shows how abnormal some of these "normal" readings are. Your report might use a cutoff of 20 µU/ml (micro-units per milliliter)[8] or higher to call a result abnormal, while the true highest normal level may be half that.

Based on research done by the Diabetes Trials Unit of the University of Oxford Centre for Diabetes, Endocrinology, and Metabolism in Great Britain, we can see how early the deadly process of insulin resistance begins. They use a tool called **HOMA**, which stands for **H**omeostatic **M**odel

---

8. In this book, I am using the units of measure conventionally found in laboratory reports in the United States. A different reporting system (SI for Système Internationale d'unités) has replaced the conventional metric system in scientific journals and is in everyday use in many other nations.

Assessment. Oxford's algorithms give a much clearer picture of the different phases of Type 2 diabetes.

For example, consider a young woman with a fasting insulin level of 19 µU/ml who also has a plasma glucose level of 89 mg/dL (milligrams per deciliter), Both of these results individually are considered normal on most laboratory reports. Yet, taken together, they show that she already has significant insulin resistance. Her receiving cells already have only about 40 percent of their normal insulin sensitivity. Her fasting glucose level remains normal, but only because her pancreas' insulin-producing beta cells are forced to overproduce about 80 percent more insulin than they should have to. There is a good chance that this woman may be slightly overweight and is developing polycystic ovary syndrome.

The additional analysis used to determine the severity of this young woman's problem required combining the results from two separate tests, her insulin level and her glucose level, both measured simultaneously. It is a good example of how using multiple tests together can often provide far more information than one test by itself. The University of Oxford made this important tool available[9] to you and your physician in a downloadable app. Bring this tool to your physician's attention since all that it requires is entering these two test results to provide a clearer picture.

2. Comprehensive metabolic chemistry panel. A chemistry panel is a predetermined group of tests done

---

9. Further information about the Oxford HOMA Calculator can be found at https://www.dtu.ox.ac.uk/homacalculator It is downloadable for free from that website.

together. Comprehensive indicates a larger (but common) group. Because these tests are highly automated, doing this large group is much faster and less costly than running each test separately.

Other tests are included in the panel but for this purpose, focus on these three results. They are your **fasting glucose**, your **liver function,** and your **kidney function.**

Your **glucose level** shows how well your blood sugar is controlled after you have fasted overnight. If it is **over 125 mg/dl** (on two consecutive occasions), it signifies diabetes. If it is **between 100 and 125**, it indicates prediabetes. If it is **less than 100**, it is supposedly normal.

However, "normal" glucose can easily be a "false negative." Although it did not reach the diagnostic threshold for diabetes, all might not be well. In the HOMA calculator example, the young woman's fasting glucose level was 89; yet, combining that reading with her insulin level, she already had significant insulin resistance. Her receiving cells had lost significant sensitivity, and her pancreas was overworked, producing extra insulin to keep her glucose level "normal."

Another issue is that when your glucose is well controlled, it should rise when you eat but return to normal two hours later. If it does not return back down, your average glucose level over time will be high; something that taking one simple reading does not spot. Your body might not be able to normalize your glucose in two hours but can bring it down with an overnight fast, which is another reason that simply checking your glucose level can produce a false negative report. Fasting blood glucose is useful information when it is abnormal. Still, a normal reading by itself does not mean you are well, which is another way to miss a diagnosis while your body is being actively harmed.

Your Liver Function can be assessed by increased levels of two enzymes in the chemistry panel. These are **AST** (Aspartate Transaminase) and **ALT** (Alanine Transaminase). If either or both exceed the normal range in the lab report, it can show your liver is inflamed. Liver inflammation can come from various causes, but the most common issue today ties into the very problems in which we are interested. Your physician will still want to check other possibilities. Today, the most likely cause of a fatty liver is associated with overweight, which is called **NASH** for **N**on-**A**lcoholic **S**teato**h**epatitis, an inflammation resulting from continued **NAFLD** or **N**on-**A**lcoholic **F**atty **L**iver **D**isease. If that condition is allowed to continue unchecked, it can progress to cirrhosis of the liver and eventual liver failure. Fortunately, unless it is in that late stage of cirrhosis, dietary metabolic change can reverse these problems. As a precaution, any time your liver is inflamed, avoid other things that might worsen inflammation. These include alcoholic beverages, the common pain reliever acetaminophen, and any other medications or toxic chemicals that could further inflame your liver.

Your Kidney Function. Your report should include **GFR** for **G**lomerular **F**iltration **R**ate, which is calculated using other tests in the panel. Anything over 59 is good and often is shown as "at least 60" or ≥60. If it is lower than 60, there is a problem, but a single test is not enough to judge this as a diagnosis of kidney failure. The report might indicate stage one,

Chapter 6: Objective Testing

two, or three kidney disease. If it is stage one, your physician is likely to schedule a repeat test. The good news is that a slight decrease in GFR often clears up on the second test, particularly if you change your dietary metabolism. Stage two or three is more serious, and your physician will explore the situation further.

3. Your High Sensitivity C-Reactive Protein. This is also known as **HS-CRP** and is a marker for inflammation. It may be found in the metabolic syndrome. However, it is not specific only to that, so infection and other forms of inflammation can also trigger it. The version of this test being used may differ from one laboratory to another, so use the normal range noted in the report.

4. Your Hemoglobin A1c is also called *glycated* and *glycosylated* hemoglobin, HbA1c, or simply **A1c**. It indirectly measures your average glucose level over the past two to three months, making it a far better way to evaluate the severity of diabetes than a single glucose reading. It is reported as the percentage of your red blood cells modified by sugar attachment during their multi-month lifetime. The report often includes a calculated second item, **E**stimated **A**verage **G**lucose or **EAG**.

A1c is very useful, but there are two reasons it occasionally provides an inaccurate reading. The test measures abnormal hemoglobin percentage, so people with a hereditary hemoglobin abnormality will get an inaccurate reading. People who have lost blood through illness or surgery will have a higher percentage of younger blood cells so that a smaller percentage will be affected by sugar exposure. If either of these conditions exists, your doctor can order a substitute test called **Serum Fructosamine**. The Fructosamine test provides information about your glucose for several weeks rather than months but is not subject to the same interference.

Although the A1c test was first developed to monitor those already diagnosed as diabetic, today it is recognized as a better screening tool than fasting blood glucose. Interpreting an A1c report can be confusing because of these two distinct purposes it serves.

When A1c is used to monitor a person taking medication for diabetes, the current recommended "normal goal" is <u>not less than 7 percent</u>. The allowance is even higher, 7.5 percent or 8 percent for older diabetics. Those percentages are considerably above what is considered normal for everyone else but have been deliberately set very high **to protect the patient from the medication itself.** When diabetic medication is used to control diabetes, it will drive blood sugar <u>too low</u> at various times.

Those medication-induced severe hypoglycemic episodes can do great harm, including brain damage from strokes, dementia, and even death. Using a higher percentage as a goal for people who are on medication is a compromise balancing the harm from diabetes and the harm from the medication itself. Conversely, those people who can bring their diabetes under control with the correct dietary metabolic change **without using any diabetic medication can set a**

Chapter 6: Objective Testing

goal within the truly normal range!

This dual-standard may trick you when you review your test report. When the A1c test first was used, the dividing line between normal and diabetes was 6 percent. Today, a result **greater than 6.5 percent** is used to define **diabetes**. That change allowed researchers to create a new category between normal and diabetic, so today, if your percentage falls **between 5.7 percent and 6.5 percent,** you are called **prediabetic**. People with values **below 5.7 percent** are considered **"normal"** by this test. Whatever names get assigned to these categories, they mean that if **your A1c is 5.7 percent or higher**, you likely have some degree of insulin resistance and its associated risks.

5. Your Lipid Profile shows the levels of cholesterol and other fat in your blood. Today, Americans are bombarded by television commercials claiming they can become healthier by asking their doctor for a certain medication. It might surprise many to learn that the United States is one of the few places in the world where this type of advertising is still legal! It uses 1950s thinking to make people believe that all cholesterol is evil.

As discussed in Chapter 3, **cholesterol is vital, necessary for life, and made within our bodies**. It is true that drugs lowering total cholesterol, when all else is equal, lower some heart disease risk for certain people, but that conclusion is based upon studying Americans who ate a typical high-sugar diet, they were likely to already have a pre-existing metabolic abnormality.

Instead, look at correcting the underlying problem. Research clearly shows that other measures in your lipid profile are far more useful than total cholesterol and will be better predictors of your future risk. Differences in levels of **High-Density** and **Low-Density Lipoproteins**, better known as **HDL** and **LDL** cholesterol (or good and bad cholesterol), are far more important. While the cholesterol particles' size is important, the amount of circulating fats, known as *triglycerides* (**TG**), is very important. The ratios between some of these components explain even more about your health risk.

Although there are expensive exotic tests offer additional predictions, the most accurate predictor of future risk is simply the **ratio of TG to HDL**, both present in a standard lipid profile. Dividing the **TG** number by the **HDL** number predicts cardiovascular risk. An answer **less than 2** predicts that you are in a **low-risk** group. "Ideal cutoff-values" may be as low as 1.62 in men and 1.18 in women. From **2 to 4,** you fall into the middle, the "**normal range**" with cardio-vascular risk increasing as the number increases; **above 4** means **higher risk**.

This science has been known for years,[10] but the influence of the drug industry is powerful. There is an axiom that when your only tool is a hammer, everything looks like a nail. Due to the availability of drugs that primarily lower total

---

10. Gasevic et al. **Clinical usefulness of lipid ratios to identify men and women with metabolic syndrome: a cross-sectional study.** *Lipids in Health & Disease* 2014, 13:159
- Debette S et al. **Plasma lipids and cerebral small vessel disease.** *Neurology* 83 November 11, 2014
- Quispe R et al. **Relationship of the triglyceride to high-density lipoprotein cholesterol (TG/HDL-C) ratio to the remainder of the lipid profile: the very large database of lipids-4 (VLDL-4) study.** *Atherosclerosis,* 2015 Sep. 242(1) doi: 10.1016/j.atherosclerosis.2015.06.057

cholesterol level, the idea that this is the best way to lower risk persists. In truth, you may not need powerful or expensive drugs to reverse cardiovascular risk and you may do a better job by eliminating the underlying causes. A high triglyceride level may mean that a high insulin level is commanding your liver to convert excessive sugar into fat. A high triglyceride level, in itself, may be a marker for insulin resistance and inflammation. Inflammation begins the process of building the plaque within your blood vessels that lead to heart disease. Cholesterol is found within that plaque, but it is essentially a building block. The underlying cause that starts the process of plaque creation is inflammation.

That inflammatory risk will rapidly improve with metabolically appropriate dietary change. As triglyceride levels fall, the ratio TG/HDL will also fall. HDL, the good cholesterol, will increase gradually over time, lowering the ratio even more. It is not unusual for this predictive ratio to fall from the highest risk, through the normal risk, and down to the lowest risk in a matter of months, all without the need for medication. As this is occurring, the reduction of chronic inflammation makes you better able to fight off disease. Work with your physician, monitoring this important predictor. Although statistical predictions cannot be a guarantee, by doing so, you will be changing your odds of staying healthy.

The remaining two tests should be done if you suspect a vitamin D deficiency.

6. Your Vitamin D level (25-Hydroxy) will quickly determine if your vitamin D level is adequate, but the current reporting labels are misleading. Generally, only levels below 20 ng/mL (nanograms per milliliter) are called "Vitamin D deficiency," while levels less than 30 ng/mL are called "Vitamin D insufficiency." These labels are based upon needs to prevent soft bones in rickets and osteomalacia.

Now that science understands that vitamin D is a powerful hormone controlling your immune system, higher levels should be called for. Inadequate vitamin D will play havoc with your immune system, on the one hand, not appropriately fighting off disease and, on the other hand, mistakenly attacking your own healthy tissue in autoimmune disease.

One authoritative guide[11] suggests that 38 ng/mL is a more appropriate cutoff for neuromuscular disorders (such as fibromyalgia and myositis) and 52 ng/mL for reducing the risk of breast cancer. Based on both published research information and clinical experience, my opinion is that maintaining a level between 60 and 80 ng/mL is an ideal goal. The next chapter will explain how to do this.

Warning: *Do not allow this level to go over 100 ng/mL. Vitamin D is a fat-soluble vitamin, which means your body stores it in fat. That allows you to build adequate levels during the summer, which carry you through the winter. Fat-soluble vitamins (A and D) are the only forms of vitamin that can reach excessive and toxic levels. In nature, your body will regulate itself and prevent excessive vitamin D levels from being formed, but people using supplements can exceed safe limits.*

---

11. Rao L., and Snyder L., editors. **Wallach's Interpretation of Diagnostic Tests 11th edition.** Walters Kluwer, Philadelphia 2021

Chapter 6: Objective Testing

7. Erythrocyte Sedimentation Rate (also known as ESR, Sed Rate, or sedimentation rate) is a very generalized measure of inflammation. It is non-specific and does not identify any particular disease. It can be very useful if elevated because it can be used as a gauge to see when therapies help the inflammation go down.

If your vitamin D level is low and your sedimentation rate is high, it might be because of an autoimmune reaction. If you begin therapy, seeing this marker returning to normal can show you this therapy is helping.

This chapter provided a recommendation for tests if you suspected you might have two significant inflammation sources, insulin resistance and low Vitamin D.

For suspected **insulin resistance**, the following tests were recommended:
   1. Fasting Insulin Level
   2. Comprehensive Metabolic Chemistry Panel
   3. High-sensitivity C-Reactive protein
   4. Hemoglobin A1c and
   5. Lipid Profile

You also learned how you and your physician could get a more accurate picture of your insulin resistance using the easily available **Oxford HOMA calculation app**.

For a suspected **low vitamin D**, I suggested these tests:
   6. Vitamin D Level (25-hydroxy) and
   7. Erythrocyte Sedimentation Rate.

Fighting Covid-19, the Unequal Opportunity Killer

This chapter provided you much detailed technical information, which I hope you are able to use. As a physician, I believe that when people understand what is happening to them, they are more likely to be able to control their own lives. If you could not get this testing done or see your physician, do not despair. Almost everything that follows in this book can guide you to becoming healthier without these complex tests. Those of you who can get this testing done will be in a stronger position since you can see what is needed and have a way to measure your improvements. Whether you had the chance to get these evaluations done or not, do not delay starting the plans that follow.

There is no way a book can provide detailed personalized guidance for you, nor can it replace your relationship with your doctor. Still, disease prevention and moving toward better health ultimately will depend on your own decisions and actions.

Chapter 7

Boosting Vitamin D

This is a quick and easy chapter, but it is important. **The best way to safely and quickly increase your Vitamin D level is by taking an adequate Vitamin D supplement.** If you have worked with your physician and know your Vitamin D level, you can safely raise it. Either you can receive a prescription for Vitamin D_2, which comes in a large dose of 50,000 iu (international units) that you take once a week for two months, or you will use over-the-counter Vitamin D_3 10,000 iu daily for two months in the form of two tiny capsules of 5,000 iu each. These are also be labeled as 125 mcg (micrograms) each. Discuss this with your physician, and be sure to re-check your blood level at the end of two months. You should then switch to a lower maintenance dose, somewhere between 2,000 and 5,000 iu of Vitamin D_3 each day. A Vitamin D supplement is inexpensive, a few cents a day at most pharmacies. I suggest over-the-counter for Vitamin D_3 for three reasons. D_3 is the natural form you make yourself. It is easier for people to take something daily than to remember to take it one day a week. It is easier to switch to a daily maintenance dose when you have already been taking Vitamin D daily.

Chapter 7: Boosting Vitamin D

When you get your re-check, how much and how fast your Vitamin D level came up will guide you and your physician in deciding whether your maintenance dose should be higher or lower. For optimum benefit, most people are best at a level between 60 ng/mL to 80 ng/mL.

Many people ask about additional Vitamin D they may be taking, perhaps from fortified food, a multivitamin, or a calcium supplement. Usually, compared to the larger amounts just discussed, these are relatively small. If you were taking them in the period you were tested, their effect has been taken into account. One exception is cod-liver oil, which was once popular in the United States and is still popular in Scandinavia. One tablespoon (about 15 mL) contains almost 2,000 iu of Vitamin D. Therefore, people taking cod-liver oil are less likely to be low in Vitamin D. Cod-liver oil use definitely should be taken into account.

What about Vitamin D in food? Most foods contain little Vitamin D, except for those fortified artificially, such as milk. The best natural sources include wild-caught dark fish such as salmon, tuna, and trout, which all contain healthy fish oils. These each have about 500 to 600 iu in a 3-ounce portion. Farm-raised fish may contain less. Pale colored fish such as tilapia contains very little fish oil by comparison. Eggs contain over 40 iu each in their yolks. However, some premium and farm eggs with darker yolks contain a bit more. Liver also contains over 40 iu in a 3-ounce portion, but muscle meat, such as chicken breast or ground beef, only has about 2 to 4 ng/mL in the same size portion. Most vegetables (except mushrooms), grains, and fruit contain none.

Increasing your sun exposure will help, but it is probably not going to be enough unless you are working outdoors. We have done so much to avoid sunlight (due to cancer fear) that getting enough sunlight is difficult. Air conditioning makes staying inside too comfortable to want to leave. Since sunlight is filtered by the sun's angle, the same amount of time spent in New York, Chicago, or Seattle results in lower exposure to ultraviolet light than in a Sunbelt city, such as Miami, Houston, or San Diego.

Your genetic makeup, which includes your skin color and how well you tan, matter considerably. This is the one area where genetic differences matter, but racial labels in the United States do little to clarify this. The racial label Black in the United States defines historic social labels and prejudices, but includes a wide range of skin color. Melanin, the color pigment in everyone's skin, protects against harmful overexposure to ultraviolet light in very sunny areas. At the same time, skin color reduces Vitamin D creation for those in regions receiving less sunlight. Comparing two people having equal portions of outdoor time, a Black person living in Seattle is extremely likely to be low in naturally produced Vitamin D, while a person of Scandinavian descent living in Miami is more likely to be at risk of severe sunburn as well as skin cancer.

You still want to avoid overexposure to the intense sunlight that can lead to higher skin cancer rates. Use the compromise advice from the experts who understand both sides. Keep your daily sunlight exposure to about half the time

Chapter 7: Boosting Vitamin D

that would give you a sunburn. That is a specific amount that is better suited to you than any fixed number of minutes or similar restrictions. Unless you are regularly working outdoors, the amount that your body can raise your Vitamin D level will be less than the amount you will get from taking a supplement. A second determinant is how well you absorb a supplement. Vitamin D is fat-soluble, which means that people who absorb fat poorly may not raise their level as quickly. This might apply to you if you have had your gall bladder removed. These differences provide a good reason to test your actual level before you start and a re-check it after two months of attempting to boost your level.

What should you do if you have not been able to get your Vitamin D tested? You need Vitamin D as much as anyone else, but use more caution. Take time to get to a higher level. Skip the loading dose and start taking over-the-counter Vitamin D_3 at between 2,000 and 5,000 iu each day. The use of this amount will not get you up to the optimal level as quickly but will still give you a decent level and should preclude any chance of your taking too much, which you were warned about in the last chapter.

What have you gained by improving your Vitamin D level? Your priority right now is building a wall to protect you from the Covid-19 virus. At this point, there have been no direct clinical trials specifically between these two items; yet experts point to secondary data that shows how effective a high Vitamin D_3 level may be. One example is a scientific paper[12]

---

12. Ilie P. et al. **The role of vitamin D in the prevention of coronavirus disease 2019 infection and mortality.** *Aging Clinical and Experimental Research* 32, 1195–1198 (2020)   DOI 10.1007/s40520-020-01570-8

comparing Vitamin D levels among people in different regions of Europe with percentages of severe cases in those regions. It claims to correlate nations with higher Vitamin D levels among their people with lower death rates from Covid-19. This makes sense for two reasons. We know that a low Vitamin D level means your immune system can't do its job against foreign invaders. We also know that sometimes low levels may be associated with autoimmune-induced inflammation. In many other pulmonary disease types, a low Vitamin D level is associated with more severe illness.[13] It is too late to increase Vitamin D when someone is critically ill. Increasing the level of Vitamin D beforehand reduces the chance of developing severe illness and many pulmonary diseases.

Zinc is discussed in the Appendix to this book on page 189. This important mineral is also associated with the function of your immune system. Since you are concerned with your immune system function, consider adding a zinc supplement when boosting your vitamin D level.

What else have you accomplished by increasing your Vitamin D level? In addition to building a wall against severe Covid-19 infection, you have created a protective barrier against a variety of diseases. These include increased resistance to pulmonary diseases (such as asthma and

---

13. Grant et al. **Evidence that Vitamin D Supplementation Could Reduce Risk of Influenza and Covid-19 Infections and Deaths.** *Nutrients* **12**: 988 (2020). DOI 10.3390/nu12040988
- Cannell et al. **Epidemic influenza and vitamin D.** *Epidemiol. Infect* **134**: 1129–1140 (2006).
- Agrawal et al. **Vitamin D and Bronchial Asthma: An Overview of Data From the Past 5 Years.** *Clinical Therapeutics* **39**(5): 917-929 (2017).
- Wu et al. **Effects of vitamin D supplementation on the outcomes of patients with pulmonary tuberculosis: a systematic review and meta-analysis.** *BMC Pulmonary Medicine* **18**:108 (2018).

Chapter 7: Boosting Vitamin D

COPD), several types of cancer, and many autoimmune disorders.

Isn't it time to push aside the makers of more costly drugs and ask the question, "Why isn't everyone being checked for Vitamin D to prevent disease?" Don't wait; first get your level tested by your doctor if you can, but **get started**.[14] Do this both to protect yourself from severe Covid-19 and help prevent or heal other chronic diseases.

---

14. Mittchell F. **Vitamin-D and Covid-19: Do deficient risk a poorer outcome?** *The Lancet Diabetes & Endocrinology* 8 (7) 570. (2020). DOI 10.1016/S2213-8587(20)30183-2

Chapter 8

Reversing Insulin Resistance

The last chapter was easy since you were able to make a small change that should have produced big results. The next step is going to be harder, but the benefits will be even greater. **Insulin resistance is a big deal**. It eats away at your health before you recognize it. Resistance to Covid-19 is why you started, but you learned that you would be protecting yourself from other serious future problems, too. Whether you are exposed to Covid-19 or not, you will be rewarded through improved day-to-day health.

Reversing insulin resistance is not hard, but uses one "dirty four-letter word." That word is *diet*. People may be scared, disgusted, or angry when they hear that word. Thousands of advice books are available on diet, with about 99 percent of them nonsense. Whether it is a country singer who offers cabbage soup or a doctor who offers magic-smelling food, it is a publishing game. Get a celebrity name on a ghost-written diet book, and truth does not matter. People who fail on the endorsed diet create a market for the next celebrity book. The same goes for "magic products." When the fad is over, it is time to sell another product or another book; use a different

Chapter 8: Reversing Insulin Resistance

celebrity endorsement, whether on television or Facebook.

The truth is, **simple dietary change does work**. That knowledge is ageless. It does not require tens of thousands of dollars in medications each year or selling of food or bariatric surgery. I have attended "informational meetings" by hucksters who soak their victims for as much as $15,000. I have also been treated to luxury dinners by people wanting to find doctors who would lease "magic machines" to sculpt away fat from desperate patients.

Real dietary change should not make anyone wealthy. People have known about dietary change for more than 2,000 years, and it still works. That truth gets obscured by the noise from hucksters, moneymakers, and pseudo-scientists who are lining their own pockets. A science of propaganda fortifies all this hucksterism and has been used and abused by governments and military dictators throughout history. When the noise gets loud enough and frequent enough, many believe it. Even those who should be skeptical go along with it. Some appear to be leaders, running ahead of the crowd, and agreeing with the latest fad, just so they do not appear ignorant.

Our own "authorities" can and do get taken in. One example of this occurred in the 1970s, but it was only a few years ago that the truths about bribery of "key scientists" came out. In the meantime, the federal government not only accepted these lies, but the government arbitrarily set a standard to convince all Americans of a supposed "truth", one claiming that low-fat dieting would improve their health. When all this became known, those same pompous agencies never admitted they were at fault. The result was a doubling of the number of people who have type II diabetes and many greatly overweight and obese. Some of these bad ideas even started over a century ago, before heart attacks were a common medical occurrence. Yet, many centuries ago, people recognized that certain diseases were caused by diet.

In Chapter 3, you learned that to get healthy; you had to relearn wrong ideas. Luckily, getting healthy does not mean following fads, eating rice cakes with kale, or ingesting strange foreign fruits. People who have come to me to overcome diabetes, overweight, and related problems are often desperate. They previously unsuccessfully tried to diet and are now worse off. Most had been miserable during the past times that they had tried to diet. Some wasted thousands of dollars buying products from hucksters. Others even tried surgery.

When I tell folks the "secret," they are skeptical before they begin. Once they start, they find that they are eating real food, sometimes for the first time in their lives, and they love it. Instead of that dreaded word "diet," they undergo a lifestyle change. They can find that enjoyable and sustainable while they feel better and are truly healthier.

Let us start with the basics. Your insulin resistance came about as a normal response to an excess of energy being taken in. It is as simple as that. Your body produces more insulin whenever it must deal with a high-energy intake that creates increased blood sugar. So far, that response is perfectly normal. It is the quantity and the frequency of these episodes that harm you. Compare those dietary excesses to going to rock concerts or working in a noisy machine shop

Chapter 8: Reversing Insulin Resistance

where the abundance of sound damages your hearing. Frequent excessive eating creates an abundance of blood sugar, which damages your body's ability to cope. Your body must respond to this extra energy you consume, and it does so, producing more and more insulin as the need dictates. As your receiving cells become overwhelmed with extra insulin, they become resistant to it. In effect, they become deaf to a normal level of insulin signal. Your body has to respond by producing even more insulin, establishing a vicious cycle.

Eventually, you have difficulty making enough insulin to keep your blood sugar down. That is usually the first point at which diabetes is typically diagnosed. In type II diabetes, at first you can still produce large amounts of your own natural insulin, but it is still not enough, because your cells have lost sensitivity to insulin. At that stage, you are not deficient in producing insulin; it is a relative insufficiency because you have become insensitive to it.

The answer, for many people, is simple. Give your body time to rest and time to restore your normal sensitivity. Once that is achieved, never go back, thinking you are now "cured." Instead, be cautious and avoid the traps that caused the problem in the first place.

That is an important distinction. Successfully treated cancer patients are cautious, calling themselves "in remission" but not cured. They remain watchful for the rest of their lives. Those who successfully conquer addiction may refer to themselves as "recovering" rather than recovered. They cannot return to their former selves without endangering their lives. They say that "You may remove a pickle from brine and wash it in fresh water, but it will never return to being a fresh cucumber." So, it is with insulin resistance. With the right diet, insulin resistance and its consequences may be reversed, but that is not a reason to stop doing the right thing. A healthy diet is a lifestyle change that should become a lifetime change. Fortunately, healthy foods are real and taste better than rice cakes and kale.

With diet comes weight-loss, for those who need it. This book is not about weight or weight loss, and yet, it is. Unwanted weight gain is a marker for the bad metabolic changes your body has gone through. Although your priority is improving your metabolism, you should expect to shed weight as you become healthier. If you start overweight, weight-loss is one way to monitor how well you are doing. The objective lab test markers of insulin resistance mean you need to visit your doctor and give blood samples, not feedback you receive every day. On the other hand, losing weight, having your clothes feel too loose, getting to shop for smaller sizes, and getting compliments from others are all clear signs of success, ones you may begin to experience frequently. Follow the plan outlined in the next chapters. As you lose insulin resistance, your body will be better able to fight Covid-19. At the same time, expect your mood to improve along with your health as you experience success and recognize that you are regaining control over your own destiny.

Chapter 9:

Diets Are Not All the Same

It is inaccurate to say that most diets are equal or that a calorie[15] is a calorie. Yet, there are outlandish claims made about diets that do not work, based on that very oversimplification *"just eat less and exercise more."* In that over-simplified theory, just the lowering energy intake of food or increasing the energy that you burn through increased activity, your body will burn off its stored energy, and you will lose weight. It is a simple and appealing theory, *but it is wrong*. It will work if you are a laboratory rat locked into a cage, but to make it work for real people, you would have to lock them up too. Your body has a complex mechanism to maintain energy balance and will persuade you to eat more. If you have tried such a diet previously to lose weight, and you were not successful, **you did not fail at dieting; your diet failed you.**

Those trying to sell a weight-loss product and hoping to look scientific can use an easy strategy. The food hucksters may conduct a study where subjects are paid to eat a

---

15. I will usually follow the US nutritional convention, by often using the word calorie to represent the scientific term kilocalorie (Kcal). 1 kcal is the energy needed to raise the temperature of 1 kilogram of water by 1° Celsius. That is a metric definition but many nations moved on to use the International Standard unit kilojoule (kJ). One calorie is equal to about 4.2 kJ.

Chapter 9: Diets Are Not All the Same

controlled diet in a locked environment. Under those conditions, they can demonstrate that almost any diet will work. If they were to open up the locked environment, I wonder how many subjects would quickly order a pizza delivery? Such "proof" has no relationship to the real world, where many factors drive what and how much people eat.

Some diets do exactly the opposite of what you want, even causing you to gain weight when you had hoped to lose weight. **The type of foods you eat can drive hunger and cravings, causing you to eat even more.** Food companies know this and have many practices, including chemical manipulation, all of which can wreak havoc with your health. These manipulations can trick your blood sugar, leading to wide swings in your insulin level, which creates insulin resistance and fuels strong hunger and cravings, leading to overeating.

The <u>worst</u> method of dieting is the low-fat diet.[16] If you reduce or eliminate fat from food but try to keep your energy levels the same, you have to increase something else. Although you can increase either protein or carbohydrate, food manufacturers generally increase carbohydrate because it is cheap. That means that a low-fat diet becomes a high-carbohydrate diet, with a high glycemic index and a high glycemic load. The result is that your blood sugar increases rapidly, which triggers your body to increase insulin in an attempt to control your blood sugar level rapidly. It may overshoot, creating a *yo-yo effect*. If so, your rapidly falling

---

16. Arumugam V, et al. **A high-glycemic meal pattern elicited increased subjective appetite sensations in overweight and obese women.** *Appetite*, 50(1-2) 215-22, March-May 2008.

blood sugar creates new hunger, making you eat more. Many people experience moderate reactive hypoglycemia, needing a mid-morning snack. How often have you heard, *"My blood sugar is low, I can't think straight until I get something to eat"*?

Ranchers and farmers have understood this for millennia since a high-carbohydrate diet is the standard way to fatten an animal going to market. Hippocrates, the revered ancient Greek physician, understood this when 2,400 years ago, he described[17] a method for losing or gaining weight. His method for gaining weight is the very method our government mistakenly recommended for good health and losing weight. Beginning in 1979, the Federal Government made low-fat dieting official government policy.[18] In doing so, they went against everything science knew about metabolism and appetite.

How is it possible that such wrong advice was ever acceptable? Chapter 3 revealed that "scientists" were secretly receiving payments from the sugar lobby to deflect their industry's criticism and falsely claim the issue was dietary fat. They claimed that Asians had very low diabetes or heart disease rates due to a high proportion of rice in their diet. They ignored the actuality, since physiologists and epidemiologists have long known that it was starvation that had reduced diabetes and insulin resistance, leading to less heart disease.

---

17. Littré MPÉ. **Du règime â suîvre pour pedre ou gagner de l'embonpoînt, in: Oeuvres Complètes D'Hippocrate, traduction nouvelle avec le texte Greg, Vol 6:** pp 76-79, Chez J.B. Baillière, Paris, 1849.

18. Public Health Service. **Promoting Health/Preventing Disease: Objectives for the Nation,** p 75, US Department of Health and Human Services, Washington, DC 1980.
• Cohen, I.A. **U.S. Health Objectives for 1990: A Maryland Evaluation,** Maryland Department of Health & Mental Hygiene, Baltimore, 1984.

Chapter 9: Diets Are Not All the Same

In China, for example, Chairman Mao's "Great Leap Forward" created a widespread famine that resulted in as many as 45 million Chinese deaths from uncontrolled starvation.

The sugar lobby was only one of several groups at fault, spreading false information about food. Another influential group was the tobacco industry. When many Americans quit cigarette smoking, the tobacco industry tried to diversify by taking control of the food industry. They maintained that control for about thirty years. They brought the knowledge they had gained while making cigarettes more addictive. As an example, Chapter 4 described that in 2006 the *Chicago Tribune* revealed a meeting a tobacco giant arranged when they bought a cookie company. Brain chemistry experts working for the cigarette industry met with food chemistry experts employed by the cookie bakery. What do you think they talked about?

With low-fat becoming Federal policy in 1979, decades of useful research that should have been done never occurred. The government was not about to fund research that would demonstrate to the public it had been wrong. Researchers looking for real answers were without funds and had to beg other sources for even the smallest studies. Those who chose to parrot the government line could get their research funded and published, advancing their careers.

Worsening the problem is the practice of allowing a revolving door between government and industry representatives. According to the Organic Consumers Organization,[19] an FDA official gave government approval to a report by the Monsanto Company purporting to support the

---

19. www.organicconsumers.org/monlink.cfm (accessed 15 August 2008)

safety of milk from cows treated with BGH (Bovine Growth Hormone), a substance which increases the milk production of dairy cows. This is a practice that has been questioned by consumers. That official was the same scientist who earlier wrote the report while she was employed by Monsanto. High-ranking federal appointees are often not experts in all the areas their agencies deal with. They may concentrate on a few special areas of concern, trusting the career bureaucrats below them to be both knowledgeable and honest. That is not always the case.

A very bright doctor, David Kessler, was Commissioner of the Food and Drug Administration (FDA) from 1990 through 1997, serving two presidents. Despite having earlier authored two books claiming to offer dietary advice, in 2018, he admitted that he did not know how he should eat or what was the cause of the obesity epidemic.[20] He said *"Something has led us to get bigger and bigger, It's coming from what we eat, and we don't fully understand it...I think we have failed in giving nutritional advice to people. If diet and exercise were the answer, we'd all do it and there wouldn't be a problem."* It is rare to see such an honest admission by a former government official.

When we move away from the very worst, those high-carbohydrate, low-fat diets, there are many diets in the middle. Understanding those diets means learning two terms, **glycemic index** and **glycemic load**. The glycemic index describes how rapidly a given food will raise your blood sugar.

---

20. Frieden J. **We Have Failed' at Giving Diet Advice, Says Former FDA Chief.** *MedPage Today* June 21, 2018.
https://www.medpagetoday.com/primarycare/dietnutrition/73631
(accessed July 29, 2020)

Chapter 9: Diets Are Not All the Same

The glycemic load dictates how long it stays up. If you eat too many carbohydrates at one time, its glycemic index forces your blood sugar to go up rapidly, but the amount you are eating determines its glycemic load. A higher glycemic load may keep it elevated for a longer time. Protein can also raise your blood sugar but generally has a lower glycemic index than carbohydrate. A large meal of protein will also increase your blood sugar but reaches that higher level at a slower pace. Think of the difference between acceleration and speed in a car. A car can accelerate up to 70 miles per hour rapidly, while a loaded truck will take longer to reach the same speed. Once there, both are traveling at the same speed.

People have devised thousands of diets over the ages. Many of these fall in the middle and are classified as good or bad, depending on what they are being used for. If you do not have to reverse insulin resistance, overweight, or type II diabetes, diets that give you adequate nutrition while still maintaining a low glycemic index and low glycemic load might be appropriate. If that is the case for you, you will find those discussed in Chapter 14, which deals with your needs once you overcome your insulin resistance. Most of us are not that lucky; you may have lose weight at the same time you overcome your insulin resistance. You will get to still get to the maintenance discussed in Chapter 14, but you'll need to reach that by taking the path outlined and lose weight as you do.

Exercise does not equal diet. Advocates of simply exercising without dietary change would have you believe that exercise alone is an effective strategy. Although exercise is often described as the key to becoming healthier, it should be considered an adjunct, adding its benefit to diet. Exercise, by itself, can make people healthier in some ways but generally does not insure weight-loss if used without effective dietary change, nor does it have the health benefits of reversing insulin resistance. Exercise can also be quite harmful when done incorrectly or overdone. Get started on an effective diet first, and then add an exercise program appropriate for you. The Appendix to this book provides some common-sense suggestions about matching exercise to your needs.

What can work? How can you find the right balance, a diet that can reverse insulin resistance and help you lose weight? Some of the characteristics of a good diet that can do this should be:

- It should curb hunger, not cause hunger.
- It should use normal foods, not resort to exotic or expensive products.
- It should make smaller portion sizes seem normal.
- It should allow enough variety so that you do not feel deprived.
- It should have a very low glycemic index and glycemic load.
- It should minimize your insulin needs, allowing your body to heal.
- It must be based upon solid physiologic principles, not wishful thinking.
- Its effectiveness should have been demonstrated for generations.

Chapter 9:   Diets Are Not All the Same

When a diet is used correctly, a truly ketogenic diet fulfills those requirements. You've probably heard that name recently, or the nickname "keto," However; many diets and products are using those names when they are not truly ketogenic. Ketogenic dieting has existed for thousands of years, although the scientific knowledge about its underlying chemistry was not understood until the 1920s. Ideas about ketogenic diets became confused with a high-protein dieting craze beginning in the 1970s,[21] and that confusion continues today with the current keto fad. The problem with the current fad is that when people try to follow bad keto advice, and it does not work, they become disillusioned. A truly ketogenic diet works very well.

Ketogenic dieting is easy to follow once you understand how ketosis works. Ketosis is a natural physical state that wild animals continue to use. It had helped people survive the cycles of nature before we went from an agricultural world to a complex industrialized society. We are now far removed from those natural cycles. Ketosis is your body's state when it needs to turn to stored fat for energy and survival. Some people will mistakenly tell you ketosis is abnormal,[22] but that is untrue. Ketosis is the method your body specifically uses to efficiently burn stored fat, your source of long-term energy efficiency.

21. Atkins RC. **Dr. Atkins' Diet Revolution: The High Calorie Way to Stay Thin Forever.** D. McKay Co; Philadelphia, 1972.

22. Ketosis is abnormal only when it is not something you are deliberately doing. As an example, if you were a type 1 diabetic and you had not taken your insulin, your blood sugar would be very high but your cells would be starving. Your body would turn to ketosis to keep you alive. Another example would be if you had a large hidden cancer that was using a lot of your blood sugar energy. Your body again would switch to ketosis to keep you alive. Finally, if you were starving, you would be in ketosis. Years ago, when we did not have better testing methods, a simple and quick urine test for ketosis could alert that something was wrong. It did not mean ketosis is bad. It is a way your body tries to survive when something else abnormal is happening.

Fighting Covid-19, the Unequal Opportunity Killer

Ounce for ounce, fat is the most efficient way your body can store long-term energy. An ounce of fat contains more than twice the energy of an ounce of either protein or carbohydrate. Stored sugar (in the form of the starch glycogen and water) is your system for short-term energy storage. Your body limits short-term storage to a few days' worth. If your body kept all of its energy as sugar, you would be so heavy that you might not have the ability to carry all that extra weight.

Since your body fat serves the important purpose of energy storage as well as other functions, fat itself is not a bad thing. The problem occurs when the fat balance gets out of hand, and you are constantly adding new fat. In earlier societies, whether agricultural or paleolithic hunter-gatherer, food was scarce during the winter. Having enough fat would provide extra energy to save your life. A youngster without a chubby-cheeked fat pad was less likely to survive a lean winter; cheek-pinching grandmothers may have been performing a valuable survival test!

In modern society, we are removed from the severity of seasonal scarcity. If you add too much fat today, your body does not automatically switch to its fat-burning mode. Today, you must make a deliberate effort to burn fat by fasting or dieting, but if you attempt to diet without going into the efficient fat-burning mode of ketosis, your body reacts as if you need more sugar. Incorrect dieting can be associated with falling or yo-yoing sugar levels that create anxiety and hunger. This is a survival signal since your body has not been told to switch energy modes. It recognizes that you are burning more energy than you are taking in, and it is telling you to eat more. Is it any

Chapter 9: Diets Are Not All the Same

wonder that dieting often results in a miserable experience and failure?

In addition to ketosis being the most efficient fat-burning mode for your body, ketosis has another benefit that is often overlooked. **Ketosis calms your brain.** When you are not in ketosis, as your brain uses energy, it signals you to eat more by creating anxiety. As an example, a high carbohydrate breakfast may cause a reactive hypoglycemic episode, when the breakfast causes your blood sugar to go up and your body's response is to release a surge of insulin which then makes your blood sugar fall rapidly. That reaction can make it difficult to concentrate if you don't have that mid-morning snack! Once you eat that sweetened pastry, you feel good again. Learning that pattern of feeling better from the sweet snack can lead people to crave sweets when upset.

Burning energy when in ketosis has the opposite effect on your brain. With an adequate supply of stored fat, ketosis has a calming effect. Fasting (one way to produce ketosis) can lead to calmness and clarity of thought, a fact that has been recognized and practiced in various cultures and religions. That calming feature is needed; without it, hibernating animals would instead be awake and roaming anxiously long before spring.

Your brain accomplishes this calming using a neurotransmitter (believed to be GABA or gamma-aminobutyric acid) with natural calming power. GABA is also increased during meditation as well from small amounts of tranquilizers and alcohol! GABA's calming action during ketosis is so powerful that either fasting or using a ketogenic diet quiets epileptic seizures. That same calming action allows people to use a ketogenic diet to eat smaller portions of food without feeling anxiety or cravings telling them to eat more. This calming action is the exact opposite of what happens when people's brains are running on sugar. It can be the key to your dietary success.

Ketosis simply means the state when ketones are circulating in your blood. Ketones are the chemical form that fat takes when your body prepares fat to be burned as energy. Your liver converts triglycerides, the fat that came out of storage, to a mixture of three chemicals, beta-hydroxybutyrate, acetoacetic acid, and acetone. Almost every cell in your body[23] can use ketones for energy.

If you have not been using ketosis for a long time, the chemical pathways in your cells may not be functioning at full efficiency. It may take a few days to adapt, but once adapted, your body will function as well as burning fat as it did burning sugar. **In addition to feeling calm, you will need far less insulin to control your blood sugar level. Reducing your need for insulin is the key to healing from insulin resistance and its associated inflammation.** Your insulin level going down will allow your insulin resistance to fade gradually, and as it does, inflammation improves. Your body can function better. This cannot prevent you from being exposed to any virus, but if you are, you will be in better shape to fight it.

---

23. The exceptions are your peripheral nerves and your red blood cells, which can only use glucose.

Chapter 9: Diets Are Not All the Same

Getting into ketosis and staying there is not difficult if you follow the plan given in Chapters 12 and 13. Once you are there, your blood sugar should fall to a level that is adequate and steady. You just have to be careful and stay in that healthy metabolic state. During this stage, don't attempt to *"cheat... just a little bit."* That would trick your body into thinking it is springtime and switch back to burning sugar, which would allow your blood sugar and insulin level to rise again. Use fat-burning as a long-term approach until you reach your goals. If you do, you will heal your insulin resistance as well as lose unwanted fat.

If you try to switch back and forth frequently between using fat and sugar, you will confuse your body. As your body burns sugar, food cravings will quickly return. Your body can then attempt to do unhealthy things to feed itself sugar. It may even dissolve down your muscle protein to create new blood sugar. Wait until you get healthier and move to a maintenance program. At that point, you can safely treat yourself to some of those "bad things" occasionally and in moderation.

Chapters 12 and 13 will provide details of how to start and follow this diet. More in-depth information can be found in my earlier book ***Dr. Cohen's New Hippocratic Diet® Guide***.[24] A Spanish language edition[25] is also available. Several useful starting recipes are included in the Appendix of this book. Additional recipes, many developed in the past by my patients,

---

24. Cohen, I.A. **Doctor Cohen's New Hippocratic Diet® Guide: How to Really Lose Weight and Beat the Obesity Epidemic.** Center for Health Information, 2008. ISBN 978-0-9820111-9-5

25. Cohen, I.A. **La Nueva Dieta HipocráticaTM del Doctor Cohen: Cómo realmente bajar de peso y vencer la epidemia de la obesidad.** Center for Health Information. 2013. ISBN 978-0-9820111-8-8

Fighting Covid-19, the Unequal Opportunity Killer
can be found in ***Cooking for the New Hippocratic Diet**®*.[26]

Be cautious when making dietary choices. Because ketogenic dieting is a hot topic today, much of the information from popular sources is wrong. Some diets and recommendations get you halfway, but a halfway point is not enough. It is easy to develop ideas that reduce carbohydrates a bit and might moderate swings in your blood sugar. **You want to do more**. Whether you are Native American, Black, Hispanic, or Caucasian--whether you have three generations of diabetes, are overweight, or have heart disease in your family, don't let other people's prejudices and stereotypes define your health. You can accomplish weight loss and improved health. If you break the mold and stick to it, you become an example for those around you and show that it can be done.

The next few paragraphs are a bit detailed but are here for background information for those who wish to know more. The diet of Hippocrates 2,400 years ago was ketogenic when evaluated by today's methods, as were some late 19th century diets[27] for weight loss and control of diabetes. Those diets were based on observation since the chemistry of ketosis was not known until the 1920s, when Doctor Wilder at the Mayo Clinic developed a therapeutic diet to control epilepsy[28] in

---

26. Cohen, I.A. **Cooking for the New Hippocratic Diet.**® Center for Health Information, 2011. ISBN 978-0-9820111-7-1

27. Ebstein, W. **Corpulence and It's Treatment on Physiological Principles, New Edition**, H. Grevel & Co.,London,1890 (first published as **Die Fettleibigkeit (Korpulenz) und ihre Behandung**, Wiesbaden, 1882).

- Ebstein W. **Über Die Lebensweise der Zuckerkranken,** Verlag Von J.F. Bergmann, Wiesbaden, 1892.

28. Wilder, R. M. **The effects of ketonemia on the course of epilepsy.** *Clinical Bulletin*, **2**:307, 1921.

Chapter 9: Diets Are Not All the Same

children. Further research by Doctor Woodyatt[29] provided precise detail about the ratio of major nutrients (fat, protein, and carbohydrate) in dietary intake needed to control ketosis, again for a therapeutic ketogenic diet. These therapeutic formulas were designed to provide a patient's full energy needs. They were not diets with the smaller portions needed for weight-reduction. The 1920s lacked the computers and programmable calculators available today, so using accurate but complex calculations was difficult. Others substituted a simplified calculation[30] for routine clinical use but warned that their simple approximation was not as accurate as the original formula. Both of these calculations were intended for a therapeutic ketogenic diet, but not for accurate use in weight loss. Today, when you find the ketogenic ratio used,[31] it can be the wrong formula and wrong circumstance. By using the simplified formula or using the therapeutic formula to evaluate weight-loss dieting, researchers will get inconsistent or misleading results. This leads to confusion as to what is and is not ketogenic. When the right formula is used appropriately, it provides a tool for a successful outcome.

The original formulas were not made for use with

---

29. Woodyatt's original formula for therapeutic dietary ketogenic ratio:
$$KR = \frac{(0.9 * f) + (0.46 * p)}{C + (0.1 * f) + (0.58 * p)}$$
Woodyatt, R.T. **Objects and method of diet adjustment in diabetes,** Archives of Internal Medicine, 1921.28(2), 125-141

30. The simplified but less accurate ketogenic ratio equation of Metcalf and Moriarity:
$$KR = f / (p + c)$$
Talbot, F.B., Metcalf, K.M., Moriarty, M.E. **A clinical study of epileptic children treated by ketogenic diet.** Boston Medical & Surgical Journal (now the New England Journal of Medicine) 196(3):89-96 (1927)

31. Ziberterrter, T., Zilberter, Y. **Ketogenic Ratio determines metabolic effects of macronutrients and prevents interpretive bias.** Frontiers in Nutrition. 5:75, 2018.

weight reduction, but today, insulin resistance and diabetes go together with weight loss. I extended Woodyatt's original 1921 formula for a therapeutic ketogenic diet to an expanded method to include non-dietary energy. That means that, once your body begins to burn its stored fat, you must calculate and take that additional fat into account to judge a diet's ability to work well. My expanded formula[32] is even more complex than Dr. Woodyatt's original equation, but once it is programmed into a computer, it makes developing diets more accurate. It interprets diet balance to determine a mixture that works.

The good news is that you do not need to use these formulas in choosing your meals. This discussion was necessary to warn you about the inaccuracies in many things you may hear or read about diets. Using a tool that allowed comparison of diet quality, it became possible to create a program for successful dietary change that has worked for many. I chose the name **New Hippocratic Diet**® to recognize that this modern plan bears a similarity to Hippocrates' observations and recommendations 2,400 years earlier.

Although this is the right diet for most people, some people should be more cautious. People who will need to talk to their physician and jointly decide when the time is right or if this is the right plan include:

1. Anyone healing from surgery or other types of trauma. Your body may need extra dietary protein to create new

---

32. This is the expanded formula to determine **Total Ketogenic Ration (TKR)**:
$$TKR = \frac{(0.1 * <e - [4 * (p + c)]>) + (0.46 * p)}{c + (0.011 * <e - [4 * (p + c)]>) + (0.58 * p)}$$
Cohen, I.A. **A method for determining total ketogenic ratio (TKR) for evaluating the ketogenic property of a weight- reduction diets**, Medical Hypotheses, 73 377-381 (2009). doi:10:1016/j.mehy.2009.03.039

Chapter 9: Diets Are Not All the Same

tissue. Talk to your doctor and wait until you have healed.

2. Anyone who is pregnant or planning to become pregnant. In the animal kingdom, many carry their young over the winter while they are in ketosis. However, we don't know enough about safety in humans and human development. We do know that high sugar levels can be harmful to you and your baby during pregnancy, but it makes more sense to deal with issues before becoming pregnant. It is also easier to become pregnant once you have followed this diet. Using this plan can help reverse PCOS, polycystic ovary syndrome, a condition that may have prevented you from becoming pregnant in the past. One caution for those who are not trying to become pregnant is that dietary healing of PCOS will increase fertility.

3. Anyone taking the drug **Lithium Carbonate** for bipolar disorder. Any dietary change can change the blood level of this drug and should be monitored by your doctor.

4. Anyone taking the drug **Warfarin** or a similar blood thinner. You may find yourself eating more green leafy vegetables, which can change the effectiveness of this drug and should be monitored by your doctor.

5. Anyone taking any other drug where your doctor is following blood levels, and where you have been warned that a dietary change could change the drug's effectiveness.

6. Anyone who has had an eating disorder such as anorexia or

Fighting Covid-19, the Unequal Opportunity Killer

bulimia in the past. You should always stay in touch with your doctor or therapist when following any diet.

7. Anyone who is currently taking any type of medication for type II diabetes or prediabetes. Medications <u>must</u> be reduced or, in some cases, stopped as soon as you start this diet. You will need to monitor your blood sugar and work with a doctor who understands what you are doing and why. This diet will be of great help to you, but you are likely to encounter dangerous hypoglycemic episodes if you attempt it without medication reduction, monitoring, and a physician's guidance.

8. Anyone who does not have control over his or her own food choices.

Certain ingredients prompt you to eat more, and you will need to learn what they are so that you can avoid them. Unfortunately, reading the label of processed foods is a game in the United States, with food companies trying to stay a step ahead of your understanding. Before you begin your diet, the next two chapters will explain the pitfalls of food selection. You can fight back by learning how to read tricky food labels, avoid dangerous additives, and buy real food products.

Chapter 10

Deadly Ingredients

Inflammation related to the diabetic spectrum of obesity and insulin resistance is more likely when you frequently consume dangerous food ingredients. Since obesity, type II diabetes and their underlying insulin resistance greatly increase your risk of dying from Covid-19, their danger to you should not be understated. In earlier days, processed food could contain obviously dangerous ingredients and contaminants. Laws and prohibitions stopped those, and today many laws and regulations protect consumers from those obviously immediately dangerous substances. The public could easily understand why arsenic did not belong in food.

Today, the problem is subtler; since manufacturers portray some harmful ingredients as innocent or even helpful. Instead of rapidly causing illness or death, they gradually create health problems and do their damage over the decades. The link of dangerous ingredients to dysfunction and disease is less obvious to the consumer. Government regulators often ignore it. These regulators should know better. The consumer may underestimate their danger, thanks to industry efforts to hide the truth. Like cigarette smoking or vaping, these food

Chapter 10: Deadly Ingredients

products are seductive, giving pleasure when first used; yet, they are just as deadly.

Avoiding these dangerous products is not always easy. Dangerous ingredients will trick you because they make bland food taste better. Some cheap substitute ingredients can imitate wholesome foods. Some have been in use for millennia, but in small amounts, unlike their massive use today. Earlier, those ingredients were too costly to be used routinely. Things have changed, so today those ingredients are cheap and plentiful. Sugar and glutamate-based flavor enhancers are two common items. Most people are familiar with sugar and may think of it as natural, perhaps even believe it is wholesome. Fewer people know about glutamate flavor-enhancers; yet, they are exposed to them constantly.

Sugar is natural, but its abundance and use today is not natural. Sugar in our bodies can be used as glucose for energy. In food, sugar may be sucrose, fructose, lactose, and others (look for names ending in "ose"). Some taste sweeter. Some differ in their glycemic index, but all can be converted to the blood sugar glucose, like many other foods. **All sugar should be thought of as sugar!**

Pure sugar was once a rare luxury,[33] extracted from sugar cane in ancient India thousands of years ago. Obesity and diabetes (prameha) followed but only among those who

---

33. Suzarta, as cited by Woodyatt. "**Disease of Metabolism**," *in A Textbook of Medicine, Fifth Edition*, Cecil & Kennedy editors) 1941.
• Kar, et al. "**Prognosis of Prameha on the basis of Insulin level**," *Ancient Science of Life*, Vol. 16(4), pp 277-83, April 1997.
• Hardy, et al. "**Ayurvedic Interventions for Diabetes Mellitus: A systematic review**," *AHRQ Technology Assessment* 41, U.S. Department of health and Human ServicesHHS, 2001.

could afford this luxury. The "secret process" spread to Persia, but sugar continued to be a scarce rare spice elsewhere. Once Islam spread to Persia, the knowledge of sugar production spread around the Mediterranean, reaching the Iberian Peninsula. Despite that, sugar remained costly in Europe, perhaps the equivalent of one-hundred times today's price!

The more widespread availability of sugar came at the expense of the indigenous people of the Western Hemisphere and individuals in Africa. The Europeans invaded and conquered the Western Hemisphere with a profit motive in mind. The Portuguese recognized that their territory in Brazil was suitable for growing sugar cane, but only if they could provide cheap labor to cultivate, harvest and process it. Portugal controlled forts on the African coast, which they converted to prisons for trading in enslaved people and began the process of imprisoning and transporting people as slaves to work their fields in the Western Hemisphere. When other European nations saw how the Portuguese were profiting, they quickly copied that economic model. Whether Spanish, English, Dutch, or French, if their territory was suitable for cane production, enslavement and transportation of Africans quickly followed. **Sugar created African slavery in the New World!**

The increase in sugar production led to greater use by those Europeans who could afford it. When the mid-19th century military conflict threatened France's sugar supply, they turned to the sugar beet as a sugar source, which could be grown locally. American-developed harvesting equipment next reduced labor costs associated with sugar beets. At the same

Chapter 10: Deadly Ingredients

time, railroads and steamships meant that sugar could be brought to market cheaply. By the beginning of the twentieth century, sugar became a cheap commodity. It provided cheap food energy for the poor. It made bland food items pleasant. As the song says, "a spoon full of sugar makes the medicine go down, in the most fantastic way."

By the beginning of the twentieth century, increases in tooth decay, diabetes, and heart disease became noticeable. Sugar had advanced from being a rare treat to being affordable as an occasional treat and finally to a common everyday food by the early twentieth century. Now, in the 21st-century, United States sugar consumption is reported to vary between 124 and 149 pounds per person a year, according to the U.S. Department of Agriculture.[34] That agency apparently does not believe its own figures, so they routinely claim there is about a one-third loss in actual consumption. They never explain the basis for this supposed loss; by inserting it into their calculations, they can claim every individual in the United States consumes *only* about two pounds of sugar each week.[35] No one seems to be able to explain how a third of all that the sugar was lost.

The Centers for Disease Control (CDC), an important government agency, finally has recently acknowledged that we eat too much sugar. Half a century after the sugar lobby paid scientists to lie about the health dangers of sugar, the CDC now recommends we cut sugar use by half, which, if followed,

---

34. https://www.ers.usda.gov/webdocs/DataFiles/53304/table50.xls?v=1034.5 accessed 8/20/20

35. https://www.ars.usda.gov/plains-area/gfnd/gfhnrc/docs/news-2012/the-question-of-sugar/ accessed 8/20/20

would still leave every person in the United States eating a pound of sugar each week.

As recently as December 29, 2020 the U.S. Department of Health and Human Services and the Department of Agriculture jointly issued new dietary guidelines for Americans. In doing so, they rejected the plan by their scientific advisory committee to reduce the "added sugar" upper limit by 40%! That scientific committee consisted of twenty outside physicians and academic experts they had appointed; yet the agency bureaucrats instead issued a statement claiming there was "not a preponderance of evidence" regarding the harm done by sugar consumption. This spin on reality is comparable to the bad old days, when the tobacco industry attempted to control the dialogue about whether cigarettes did any harm.

One estimate shows that **we Americans eat about twenty-five times as much sugar as we did at the time of the American Revolution**. Another U.S. Department of Agriculture estimate shows that we eat about twenty-one times as much sugar than we did in 1822. **Either way, Americans today eat many times the amount of sugar consumed in the past**.

Added flavor-enhancers are a newer threat. If you need to reverse insulin resistance or lose unwanted weight, you must avoid these whenever possible. Don't think that flavor-enhancers are some sort of spice. Spices have a taste or a fragrance of their own, which may complement the taste of food. Flavor enhancers have no inherent taste. Their role is to boost your nervous system's taste pathways by amplifying whatever other flavors may be present, whether those flavors

Chapter 10: Deadly Ingredients

are real or artificial.

MSG, which stands for **monosodium glutamate,** is the prototype of all the glutamate flavor-enhancers. Anyone who does not want to overeat should avoid it. Controversy about MSG has existed for years[36], but not about its most important role. The controversy about MSG deals with toxic reactions of two kinds, the short-term "Chinese restaurant syndrome",[37] and the long-term potential for neurologic damage with increased rates of several neurologic diseases.

Although these are very important discussions, the immediate harm from MSG is from overeating! **The sole reason that food processors add MSG to their products is to make those foods taste better.** By doing so, people will tend to eat a little more. "Just eating one" of a tasty snack may seem difficult. Animal models have shown us this for over half a century. Add MSG to the food of a group of rats, and they will eat more, rapidly become obese, and develop diabetes. MSG is a powerful flavor-enhancer that can make old and stale food tastes fresh and flavorful.

Simply put, MSG works to make bland food flavorful by turning up the volume in our taste buds. A little MSG is found in nature, but in ancient times people came across ways to produce special flavor-enhancers despite knowing nothing

---

36. Schwartz GR. **In Bad Taste: The MSG Syndrome,** 1988, Santa Fe, Health Press.

37. Zautcke JL. et al. **Chinese restaurant syndrome: a review.** *Ann Emerg Med.* 1986 Oct;15(10):1210-3.
 Although emergency room physicians first described the "Chinese Restaurant Syndrome" decades ago, more recent publications imply that it does not exist. There is ample evidence from the past, when susceptible individuals may have encountered MSG mostly in Asian restaurants. Today, MSG is everywhere and people are frequently exposed to it. This current background of constant exposure makes it more difficult to relate such reactions to specific foods or events.

about the underlying chemistry involved. In 1908, a Japanese chemist, Professor Kikunae Ikeda, discovered the key. It was the chemical MSG that caused those expensive flavor-enhancers to work. He then developed ways to mass-produce pure MSG inexpensively.

Before Professor Ikeda, strong doses of flavor enhancers were too expensive to be used routinely. Synthetically produced pure MSG changed everything and is now used around the world. Long before Ikeda, ancient Roman cooks[38] learned to ferment rotting fish, creating an additive that made everything delicious. Known as *garum* or *liquamen*, it was likely an ingredient in exotic Roman feasts for the wealthy. Food was supposedly so tasty that people would go into a special room to vomit and make room for the next course! Other cultures also used similar fermented fish sauce. The Romans may have learned of it from the Greeks. In Asia, Thailand, Vietnam, and certain Chinese coastal areas have a history of using a similar product.[39]

In later times, the Europeans developed sauces such as Worcestershire with fermented fish, while the Chinese learned to ferment soybeans for a similar purpose. Beginning in 1909, as Ikeda's inexpensive MSG became available throughout Asia, it brought fame[40] to its inventor, with the Japanese government now recognizing him as one of Japan's ten most important inventors. MSG became a cheap

---

38. Tannahill R. **Food in History.** 1988, New York, Three Rivers Press.

39. Wikepedia. **Fish Sauce.** https://en.wikipedia.org/wiki/Fish_Sauce (accessed 8/11/2020)

40. https://web.archive.org/web/20071102064825/http://www.jpo.go.jp:80/seido_e/rekishi_e/kikunae_ikeda.htm   (accessed 12/24/2020)

115

Chapter 10: Deadly Ingredients

commodity, used largely by the Asian population. The rest of the world did not pay much attention to MSG until after World War II, when Americans in Asia noticed how some Japanese items tasted more flavorful than their American equivalents.

As American food companies woke up to this supposed "miracle of chemistry", they began to add MSG to their products. It was deliberately popularized through cookbooks, advising homemakers to add a teaspoon of MSG to all their dishes. However, by the mid-1960s, warnings about MSG toxicity were beginning to be heard. Consumers became alarmed, and MSG became a dirty word. Since then, the food industry has played a cat-and-mouse game with the public. The use of MSG in processed food continues to grow unabated, but it is often disguised so that the consumer is not aware of its presence.

The food-processing industry's efforts to cloud the issue are reminiscent of earlier efforts when the tobacco industry was trying to pretend that tobacco was not harmful. Apologist scientists on the food-industry payroll continue to say that MSG is not harmful. They are better funded than those consumers, researchers, and physicians trying to spread the alarm. Public relations efforts include industry-bankrolled groups, which purport to represent consumers' food safety concerns but exist to claim that medical evidence condemning MSG is inconclusive.

Over thirty years ago, the giant tobacco companies realized that fewer people were smoking and so they diversified by buying control of food companies in the United States, which they held for several decades. Not surprisingly, the food industry now uses tactics similar to those that had worked successfully for so many years with cigarettes. Although toxicologists and consumer advocates are attempting to alert the public about toxicity issues, those public concerns continue to be vigorously denied by the food industry.

Despite all that ongoing controversy, that is not my primary reason for warning you about these chemical flavor-enhancers. **The most important reason for avoiding flavor-enhancers is the same reason that causes food companies to use them. Added flavor-enhancers work too well, making food falsely tasty and encouraging overeating. By doing their job so well, they accelerate the epidemic of overeating, causing insulin resistance, overweight, and diabetes.**

Food scientists have known about this linkage for years. Animal research beginning in the 1960s showed adding MSG to food caused animals to eat more, gain weight, and eventually become diabetic. Further experiments showed that after the MSG-fed animals had eaten more and gained weight, stopping the MSG did not immediately stop their overeating. The animals continued to eat more and gain weight for months.

Scientists who research diabetes have learned that if they need diabetic rats for an experiment, all they have to do is give the rats an injection of concentrated MSG one time. That single high dose is enough to produce Type 2 diabetes. This one issue should be enough to influence anyone trying to protect themselves or those around them. **Knowing that MSG can lead you to overeat should be reason enough to avoid it.**

Chapter 10: Deadly Ingredients

Saying *"avoid MSG"* is easy, but doing it is hard work in the United States. The term "added flavor-enhancers" is broader than simply saying MSG since the food industry has gone to great lengths to hide MSG. When physicians and consumers became alarmed at the possible toxicity of MSG, the industry began a four-pronged approach to allow them to keep adding it to food:

1. The companies feigned concern and agreed to remove MSG from baby food voluntarily. The companies did this to pacify outraged consumers who had realized that developing infants were being exposed to MSG. By removing MSG from baby food, the companies avoided stricter government regulation or an outright ban.

2. The companies hid MSG from view by developing "clean" additives. *Clean* is industry jargon for *hidden*. **Clean does not mean free of MSG; it means just the opposite.** Loose FDA regulation only requires showing MSG on the label if it has been purified. If it is manufactured, but the final step of purification is skipped, it can be labeled by something that shows what went into it. Since Ikeda and others developed many ways that MSG can be manufactured, they have various names to use in the United States. Some sound wholesome, such as "vegetable broth" or "yeast extract." Others, such as "hydrolyzed soy protein," are just mystifying to the consumer. The Appendix at the back of this book provides a list of some of these "hidden" names for MSG. Sometimes food companies even go as far as boldly stating, *"No added MSG,"* often followed by an asterisk leading to a very small print footnote saying *"except for the MSG, which naturally occurs in*

hydrolyzed soy protein." In case you were wondering, hydrolyzed soy protein is an intermediate product produced in some of the many manufacturing processes for MSG.

Because the European Union consumers have to deal with language barriers, they are protected by a series of code numbers. A European label must carry a code from E620 to E629 for any form of glutamate flavor-enhancer and the entire range of E600 through E699 is reserved for chemical flavor enhancers. If the consumer cares to look, the information is right there.

3. The food companies developed a public relations campaign, which included:

    a. Influencing the Food and Drug Administration (FDA) to officially maintain that MSG is "generally recognized as safe" and comparable to salt, pepper, vinegar, and baking powder.[41]

    b. Using the discovery of a "umami" (Japanese for "tasty") receptor is used by MSG, to publicize the idea that food additives are "natural and safe." This logic is akin to claiming that since the powerful and dangerous narcotic Fentanyl uses our brain's receptors for endorphins, Fentanyl must be natural and safe and so drug addiction must be a myth!

    c. A Japanese chemical company recently began a $10,000,000 three-year campaign[42] in the

---

41. Code of Federal Regulations, Title 21, Part 182, Subpart A. (e-CFR as of 8/10/2020)

42. Davis R. **Rescuing MSG's Unsavory Reputation.** *Wall Street Journal* April 27, 2019, Page B2

Chapter 10: Deadly Ingredients

United States encouraging food writers to once again sing the praises of MSG or umami. Their stated goal is to make Americans believe that their additive is safe and natural. This campaign is an echo of another chemical company's 1960s supermarket cookbook campaign, where every recipe provided contained a teaspoon of MSG.

4. Food companies unsuccessfully attempted to immunize themselves from lawsuits by:

    a. Attempting to have a federal law passed that would exempt food producers from lawsuits related to obesity

    b. Agreeing in 2006 to a settlement in a class-action suit brought by a group of attorneys for purportedly participating in MSG price-fixing that would give money to any state signing on but which would prevent future suits against any of the MSG manufacturers by citizens of those states **for any reason**[43]. The Attorneys General of about half the states happily agreed to receive a few million dollars for each of their state treasuries. Fortunately, the presiding federal judge saw through the ruse and eliminated the provision preventing future lawsuits.

---

43. The proposed settlement of the class-action MSG suit known as *Eugene Higgins versus Archer Daniels Midland Co.* dated March 20, 2006 was filed in the Second Judicial District Court of New Mexico. Although the suit was purportedly about MSG price-fixing, the proposed settlement included a **"covenant not to sue," which prohibited any suit by consumers against the MSG producers <u>for any reason</u> related to MSG or similar flavor enhancers**. The final settlement, fortunately, limited this prohibition to the price-fixing question. www.msgindirectsettlement.com (accessed 27 June 2006)

Fighting Covid-19, the Unequal Opportunity Killer

What is this mysterious group of chemicals, and how do they work? Glutamate or glutamic acid is a common amino acid, one of the building blocks of protein throughout nature. Whenever you eat proteins, whether that protein is from an animal or vegetable source, your digestive system breaks the proteins down into amino acids. Your body might then use those amino acids as building blocks to create new cells or break it down further and send it either into the carbohydrate or fat pathway for energy. It also might use it as a neurotransmitter, sending signals within pathways of the brain.

Glutamate is used as a common neurotransmitter, which means it is a nervous-system signaling chemical in many important brain pathways. Glutamate is found in the neural pathways dealing with taste. Attach an atom of sodium to it, and you create Monosodium Glutamate or MSG. How does that modified version of glutamate react with all the natural glutamate receptors in many diverse parts of the brain?

MSG triggers taste receptors as soon as the food containing it reaches our mouths. In addition to the taste-receptor trigger, we do not know what other effects it may have. It seems that MSG can also pass directly into our bodies through the tissues of our mouth, skipping much of the process of digestion. Since glutamate is used throughout our brain, does MSG also alter anything else? That is an unanswered question.

Various normal cooking or processing methods may modify or break down minuscule amounts of protein in normal food, but, for the most part, amino acids are not separated and freed up until the protein we eat is broken down in our digestive

Chapter 10: Deadly Ingredients

process. In contrast, the world consumption of manufactured MSG was estimated at 3.26 million tons in 2018. If that estimate is correct and distributed evenly, this is about one and a quarter pounds annually for every person on earth. It is more likely that our share is even higher since the American diet is now so high in processed food.

Since glutamate is a neurotransmitter sending signals between nerve cells in our brain, can cells in other pathways be falsely stimulated by this modified glutamate MSG? This possible false stimulation is important. **A chemical that modifies the function of a body organ (in this case, your brain) is a drug.** Some scientists not employed by the food industry worry about the toxic consequences of MSG. They worry that MSG may overstimulate other glutamate-dependent nerve cells. That theory, the *excitotoxin hypothesis*,[44] asks whether such overloaded cells suffer long-term damage. Does the increase in the number of people afflicted with neurologic disease (such as ALS, Parkinson's, or Alzheimer's) have anything to do with this?

Yet, for the purpose of controlling your diet to protect yourself, those important questions should not matter. The well-accepted point is that the addition of chemical flavor-enhancing additives does influence what and how much you eat. As the food industry has added such influencers to more products, you become their victim. **Avoid MSG and other flavor-enhancers simply because they are diet-busters.** Whether or not you become exposed to Covid-19, these changes in your diet will help protect you from having to deal with the spectrum of type II diabetes and its related complications in the future.

---

44. Blaylock R.L. ***Excitotoxins: The Taste that Kills***, 1994, Santa Fe, Health Press.

Chapter 11

Labels, Labels, Labels

You cannot protect yourself by changing your diet unless you understand what you are actually eating. Even if you are not planning to change your diet, you may be surprised to learn new things about what you are eating. Honest labeling is consumer protection, but squeezing the truth from labels in the United States can be frustrating and time-consuming. Long before people relied on prepared foods, a common form of cheating was through dishonest weights and measures,[45] a practice even mentioned in the Bible. Food adulteration came later, as people grew less of their own food. Great Britain passed its first Food Adulteration Act in 1860. The United States was later, passing our first national Pure Food and Drug Act into law in 1906 when Teddy Roosevelt was President.

Honest labeling, mandated by that 1906 law, is powerful by itself. At the time, millions of women had become addicted to remedies sold for "female complaints." Those remedies had highly addictive combinations of drugs such as opium, cocaine, and alcohol, but the users had no idea of their contents.

---

45. **Deuteronomy 25** "You shall not have in your house alternate measures, a larger and a smaller. You must have completely honest weights and completely honest measures... everyone who deals dishonestly, is abhorrent ..."

Chapter 11: Labels, Labels, Labels

Although they might relieve symptoms, their addictive nature made people feel worse if they stopped. Simply letting the user know that they were feeling ill from the "remedy" itself was enough. The truth was highly effective in stopping the epidemic from hidden narcotics. Once women realized what was in those potions, they stopped becoming victims. As sales plummeted, manufacturers had to change their formulas or go out of business.

You would think that laws and regulations are even stronger over a century later, but it is not so. While today's laws and regulations are numerous and far more complex, they are not stronger. Instead, their complexity hides simple truths. Exemptions, loopholes, and definitions protect the manufacturer from the charge of adulteration, allowing a distorted picture of what a product truly contains. Consumers who want to understand what they are eating are left in the dark, which is why this chapter will try to shed some light on this mystery.

Labeling standards follow federal law and regulation. When states attempt more stringent controls, federal agencies block them. Using the "Interstate Commerce Clause" of the Constitution, the federal government claims the sole power to regulate most products and block states from imposing stricter standards.

Industry sometimes get laws passed, which block both federal and state regulators. The US Food and Drug Administration (FDA) was once over-zealous, even prosecuting a physician for recommending the health benefits of vegetable oil! Not anymore, for in the 1990s, a federal law was enacted,

Fighting Covid-19, the Unequal Opportunity Killer

which prevents regulation of over-the-counter medications if they are instead classified as "nutritional supplements." Despite this, while the federal government does nothing when some of these are bogus, the federal law blocks states from stepping in to protect their citizens.

Some supplements are useful and healthy; some do nothing except take your money, but a few are dangerous. The FDA waits; doing nothing about a "nutritional supplement" until *after* it has harmed people. The supplement industry now boasts an economic impact of $122 billion per year and donates generously to political campaigns. The best way to protect yourself is to avoid any item when the praise for that product stems from those selling the product.

The FDA is not the only agency controlling labeling. The Department of Agriculture (USDA) writes regulations for labeling meat and poultry. A separate division of the USDA writes the standards for labels for eggs. The Treasury Department controls alcoholic beverage labels. One agency is bad enough, but four competing ones obscure your understanding of what you eat.

Let's start with the FDA because the majority of processed foods have labels following their regulations. Even there, it gets tricky. Buy prepackaged processed food in your supermarket, and it will have a required label. Purchase the same product at the delicatessen counter, and it is unlabeled. The label was on the bulk item, but you do not get to read it when they slice or serve your purchased portion.

The label has three parts. The front of the label is supposed to be truthful. However, "**puffery**" is allowed. It can

125

Chapter 11: Labels, Labels, Labels

claim that something is good or better without specifics. The FDA is supposed to prevent false health claims but allows many which are craftily worded. Look at oatmeal. The label might say oatmeal lowers cholesterol, which is truthful but only by a few points. However, it may next go on to claim it is "*heart-healthy.*" Since much oatmeal comes in packages loaded with sugar, this is a questionable claim. All that extra sugar has the opposite effect, leading to insulin resistance, inflammation, and increased heart disease.

The exact name of the product can be important, as some names are regulated. A mayonnaise called "Real mayonnaise" must contain certain minimum amounts of oil and eggs. If it has a different name, such as "Spread" or "Low-Fat Mayonnaise," it is a look-alike imitation of real mayonnaise.

Some names are not controlled at all and are not to be trusted. Real natural peanut butter is made from ground roasted peanuts. However, most peanut butter sold is made by extracting the valuable peanut oil first, then substituting a cheap oil in its place and adding sugar. It can still be called real or natural.

Puffery allows labels to emphasize expensive ingredients that are almost non-existent. People may pay double the price for mayonnaise touted as olive-oil mayonnaise. Read the label carefully, and you may find it is mostly soybean oil mayonnaise, with a small touch of olive oil listed as one of the last ingredients.

The line between puffery and what some might call lying is very thin. Beef jerky is a popular snack food. One brand claims **"No Added MSG **"** in large print on the front. The double asterisks lead to a small footnote on the back, which reads "**EXCEPT FOR THAT WHICH NATURALLY OCCURS IN HYDROLYZED CORN AND SOY PROTEIN.**" In plain English, this means **no MSG added except for that MSG we added in another form**. This is perfectly legal under labeling regulations.

Stay with this same product to see its *Ingredients List*, found on the back. The dictionary tells us jerky is *"meat, especially beef, that has been cut in strips and preserved by drying in the sun."* That sounds like wholesome outdoorsy food, but the actual ingredients in this particular product tell a different tale.

The ingredients list is supposed to show ingredients in ascending order of weight, but this is easy to get around. Split an ingredient into slightly different forms, and the manufacturer may list each separately, pushing each further down the list. Here, in boldface, are the actual ingredients with my comments in italics:

INGREDIENTS: *The list always starts with the word ingredients.*

BEEF, *You would expect beef to be the dominant ingredient, but is it? It is made from ground beef mixed with other ingredients and molded to look like cut and dried strips.*

CORN SYRUP SOLIDS, *The* **first sugar** *listed, corn syrup is a liquid sugar made by processing the starches in corn. It has been dried to a solid form.*

DEXTROSE, *The* **second sugar** *is chemically like the last one. Dextrose is also the same as glucose, your blood*

Chapter 11: Labels, Labels, Labels

sugar.

HYDROLYZED CORN AND SOY PROTEIN. *This is Monosodium Glutamate (MSG), which has been manufactured but has not been purified, allowing it to be called something else in the United States. In Europe, it would be identified by an "E-code."*

SALT,

NATURAL SMOKE FLAVOR, *Smoke from material-burning, but other ingredients may be added and not listed.*

The word "natural" does not mean what it seems. Whether it relates to the product it is in or not, any substance in nature is allowed to be called natural. Until recently, a product with a red color could contain red dye from crushed cochineal bugs, yet the label would list it as natural color. Today, this product is still allowed. It is now labeled "carmine" but does not mention crushed insects.

FLAVORINGS, *This can be virtually any form of chemical flavoring.*

WATER,

SUGAR, *This is the* **third sugar** *listed. It might be sucrose, the common table sugar from beets or some other form of sugar.*

SODIUM ERYTHORBATE. *This is an anti-oxidant to help preserve the color while it speeds the curing process of nitrite.*

CARAMEL COLOR. *This ingredient also helps it to resemble meat more closely.*

SODIUM NITRITE. *This controversial curing agent is found in processed meat products. It prevents deadly bacteria from spoiling the meat. However, too much nitrite is also dangerous. Nitrites break down into carcinogenic nitrosamines, possibly causing stomach cancer. Some people are aware of this and try to totally avoid foods containing nitrites. Manufacturers sometimes substitute celery seed extract, which contains the same chemical but gets the word "nitrite" off the label. This trick is called a "clean label" by the food industry.*

The lesson here is to prefer foods with shorter ingredient lists. Generally, the purer the food, the fewer the number of ingredients. Longer lists may spell trouble. Look for hidden forms of MSG and be suspicious of ingredients you do not recognize. The government allows different names for the same ingredient, so it is tricky. Be suspicious; even if you recognize the names of every item, you may want to question why each is there. The strategy of avoiding ingredients you do not understand may have you avoiding some innocent ingredients but will prevent many mistakes.

Despite all these issues, you should become quite positive about shopping. Once you recognize and begin using real food, you will discover not only is it better for you; it tastes better too. Shopping will take more time at first, but once you find products you like, it becomes quicker and easier. Just be prepared for a long outing the first time or two that you go shopping. You will be reading many labels.

Next, look at the familiar "**Nutrition Facts**" box. Review it even if you believe you are familiar with it since some items have changed recently.

Chapter 11: Labels, Labels, Labels

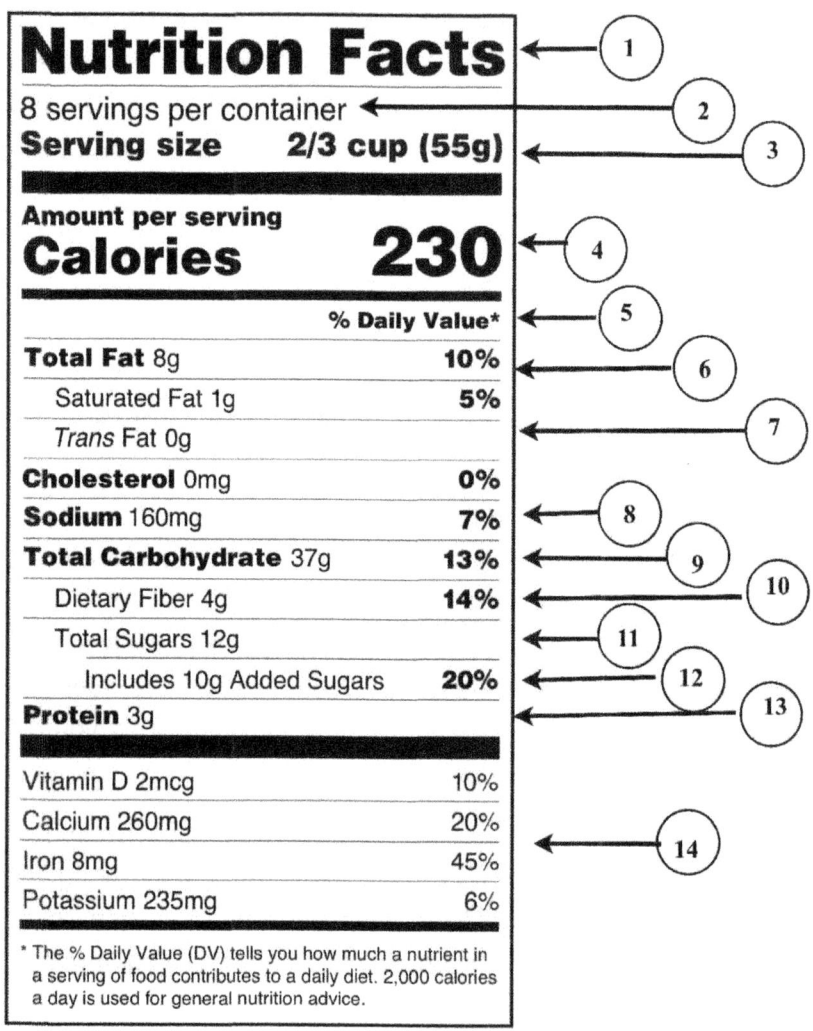

1. The heading **Nutrition Facts** is in large bold print. Smaller packages provide the same information in a textual format.

2. **Servings per container** shows how many servings are in this package. Be careful; some items describe more

portions than are reasonable, allowing the manufacturer to imply lower calorie counts.

3. The next line is **Serving Size**. Pay close attention since this size drives all the other numbers. If your serving is different, you may have to recalculate the amounts given for the serving size you use.

As you move down to the individual nutrients, note that (unlike Europe) fractional amounts are not displayed so that it may appear that an item is not present. A "sugar-free" sweetener might contain small amounts of sugar as a *flowing agent* to help it dissolve. The listing may say zero grams of sugar; yet, the ingredients list shows that dextrose, a sugar, is the first ingredient listed!

4. Calories are listed next, showing the total calories per serving. It is useful if you are tracking calories. It may overstate the case if the product contains non-absorbable energy.[46]

5. % Daily Value is a suggested recommendation you should not use. It stems from the 1940s belief that American adults should eat at least 2,000 calories each day. Because people live differently today, this is too much energy for many, causing them to gain weight dangerously.

6. Total fat is a major nutrient category and is very important. Use the grams of total fat for your diet. The subheading showing how much is Saturated Fat is a leftover warning from the old "fat-is-bad campaign."

---

46. Calories are actually measured by the heat generated when an item is burned in a furnace, called a "bomb calorimeter." Fibers that you can not digest, such as cellulose, will burn and are included, although you receive no energy from them.

Chapter 11: Labels, Labels, Labels

7.*Trans* Fat is <u>always bad</u> and should be avoided. It started as real fat but was hydrogenated, converted to an artificial form that your body handles poorly. Now recognized as bad, only a few years back, the government and the food industry claimed products high in trans fat, such as margarine, were healthy and encouraged their use.

8. Sodium is not just from salt. Excess sodium should be avoided by people who have a medical reason to do so, but other people may harm themselves by avoiding sodium. Excessive amounts of sodium in processed food often comes from MSG in one of its forms. If you see a lot of sodium listed, check ingredients carefully to see if it contains MSG or a similar flavor enhancer. By avoiding the artificial flavor-enhancing chemicals, you are avoiding that extra sodium.

9. Total Carbohydrate is also a major nutrient. It is the sum of all starches and sugars, as well as certain indigestible elements. Use this number in grams when planning your diet. You may first have to make adjustments for indigestible elements, as explained below.

10. Dietary Fiber is important but confusing. Fiber is good for you, helping your digestive tract function normally. Since certain plant material is not digested, its calories and grams of carbohydrate should not count. They are listed as energy only because of the measurement by physical burning, discussed earlier. Since you do not absorb this energy subtract these grams from the count of total carbohydrates.

11. Total sugars are a part of total carbohydrates. They were not nearly as high in human diets until the last century and a half. The other major energy component of total carbohydrate (not listed) is starch, or complex carbohydrates, which still break down to sugar. Sugars, called simple carbohydrates, will convert to your blood sugar glucose. Starches may take slightly longer to raise blood sugar, but they, too, all become sugar.

12. Added sugars are a new item in this list. Their number is already included in the total sugars figure, but it is useful to see how much additional sugar goes into foods already high in sugar. Some of these added sugars may sound natural, such as adding fruit juice concentrate purely for its sugar, but when added this way, they are being used unnaturally.

12-A. Another category, not shown in this picture but sometimes listed next, is **Sugar Alcohol**, which can alternatively be listed as an actual name of sugar alcohol, such as *Sorbitol*. Sugar alcohol, despite the name, is not related to beverage alcohol. Instead, it is a modified form of sugar used in some diet candies and confections. Although it tastes like sugar, the modification means it is not easily absorbed. The front of the label may show a number labeled **Net Carbs,** where the sugar alcohol carbohydrates have been subtracted from the total carbohydrates. You may also want to subtract the sugar alcohol number from total carbohydrate yourself, but be careful. If you eat much of this, the bacteria in your gut will break it down, changing it so that some sugar is absorbed. A little bit, such as in chewing gum, may work, but large amounts encourage the growth of gut bacteria. This will not only cause sugar absorption but also lead to gas and diarrhea!

13. Protein is the last major nutrient group. People

Chapter 11: Labels, Labels, Labels

need moderate amounts of protein in their diet. Growing children, pregnant women, people recovering from injury or doing strenuous muscle building may require more than average. Protein gets broken down into amino acids, which become the building blocks of new proteins, replacing worn-out cells and building new ones. In developed nations, people eat more protein than is needed. When they do, protein becomes an indirect source of energy. Excess amino acids are used as energy, entering energy pathways of both sugar and fat. They are roughly equally divided between these pathways.

That means protein can increase blood sugar, but it increases gradually and over a longer period. A high-protein meal will have a lower glycemic index, raising your blood sugar levels more slowly than a high-carbohydrate meal. However, it still raises your average blood sugar over some time, meaning it may have a high glycemic load, as explained in Chapter 9.

As you move to the perimeter of your local supermarket, things appear simpler. The supposedly fresh meat and poultry do not have the same complex labels but may still be highly processed. The agency regulating labels for meat and poultry is the USDA--the same agency also responsible for protecting and helping the agricultural industry. That once meant helping the farmers and ranchers produce our food, but today they are more protective of the middlemen, the food processing companies. Those middlemen are dominated by distant ownership, particularly giant meat industry corporations based in China and Brazil. Many American ranchers and farmers are under contract to those distant owners.

Way back in 1906, Upton Sinclair published *The Jungle*,

Fighting Covid-19, the Unequal Opportunity Killer

a famous book that exposed both the horrible sanitary conditions and the horrible working conditions in the meatpacking industry of Chicago. Public outrage brought about the industry's first regulation; yet, today, meat processing is more centralized than ever. When you purchase meat for home cooking, you may believe it is as natural as meat your great-grandmother cooked, but it is not.

The USDA allows alterations that can make your steak or chicken as unnatural as processed food in a can. At one time, the path from farm to table was more direct. Even in large cities, the butchers could transport cattle transported to a wholesale slaughterhouse. Fresh hanging meat, often a quarter of the animal, might reach a neighborhood butcher shop the same day. The butcher would cut the hanging meat into the familiar steaks, chops, and roasts, often as the customer waited. The meat you bought at a butcher was truly fresh. That has changed in most industrialized countries. Today, most meat-processing takes place in massive factories, far from the view of most consumers.

Instead of hanging meat, today's supermarket meat-cutters receive portions already separated into sections for final cutting, sealed in plastic and packed in cardboard boxes. Some supermarkets eliminate even this final step by having their meat products precut and packaged at the factory for retail sale. They employ no butchers or meat-cutters, just clerks wearing white butchers' robes to unpack the boxes.

A truly fresh product is long gone for most of us. Don't be fooled by the word "fresh." The USDA has redefined both the English and basic physics for us and placed their language

Chapter 11: Labels, Labels, Labels

into federal regulations. In their newspeak parlance, a food processor can call a food "fresh" if it was never below 26 degrees Fahrenheit.[47] If you are checking the weather and heard that temperature, you would understand that meant six degrees below freezing, the temperature at which water freezes at sea level. Even stranger, they can call a product "never frozen" if it has never gone below zero degrees Fahrenheit!

Worse than that are the ways that a seemingly normal piece of meat can be modified and still appear wholesome. Have you ever noticed that strange substances seem to drip out of your meat when you cook it? A process using a multi-needle injecting machine is used to treat many types of meat. It can be used for beef, pork, and poultry. One estimate is that 90 percent of pork has been treated by injection. As the meat travels down a mechanized conveyor, devices with multiple needles press into the meat and spray an unknown liquid at high pressure directly into the inside of the meat. This invention has existed for several decades, and its use continues to grow. The actual contents injected are unknown to the consumer, thanks to USDA definitions benefitting the food industry. The Center for Science in the Public Interest tried for years to get the USDA to require information about substances injected into meat. The only result is that some packages now show "_ percent retained water" in the fine print. They do not tell you what else there is in this fluid. Ground-up trimmings, chemicals for flavoring, coloring and preservation, water to increase

---

47. United States Department of Agriculture, Food Safety and Inspection Service, Last Modified Jun 25, 2013.
https://www.fsis.usda.gov/wps/portal/fsis/topics/regulatory-compliance/labeling/claims-guidance/fresh-not-frozen-and-similar-terms (accessed 9/19/2020)

weight, and who knows what else. Carbon monoxide may also be added to the air in the package, helping to keep it looking red long after it was cut.

Even those meager and misleading bits of information are only present when meats are factory-packaged for retail sale. Poultry and hams often contain that information, but meat products that arrive in bulk may not. When information does exist, compare brands. One brand of ham may have 2 percent retained fluid, while another has 15 percent. Air-chilled chicken may have none, while others may be 10 percent. When products lack information, learn by experience. Supermarket chains buy their meat from different processors; some do minimal adulteration while others may do more. Look for odd things that come out of your meat when you cook it and rely on your taste to recognize better quality.

Evaluating eggs is simpler. In the mid-20th century, eggs were considered wholesome and nutritious, with recommendations that Americans eat an egg every day. That changed when the sugar industry set out to demonize dietary cholesterol and fat. The government then advocated avoiding eggs, and many people did. Now, the pendulum has swung again, with eggs once again recognized as a wholesome and nutritious food. Egg yolks contain a healthy balance of fat to nurture a growing chick embryo, while egg whites contain protein.

Mass production economies resulted in eggs of varying quality, depending upon how the hens are fed. If you are using an egg in a recipe, you might not notice any difference, but if you are cooking it for breakfast, it will be more apparent. When

Chapter 11: Labels, Labels, Labels

hens are raised to produce better eggs, you will see darker, better-looking yolks. One way to get this is to spend more on feed, which you can see with some premium brands. You can tell the difference before purchasing because the best eggs will have more fat listed. Both the cheap eggs and the best ones are healthy, but you will notice the difference when using the better ones.

Do not be fooled by USDA-approved names "cage-free" and "free-range." These sound very natural as if hens were roaming free in the pasture, but that is not the case. Instead, if you are lucky enough to have a farmers' market nearby, you may find what some call pasture-raised eggs. Small producers may allow their hens to eat naturally with true outdoor roaming and freedom.

All eggs are healthy when cooked properly, but undercooked eggs can pose a serious health risk. They are more of a health risk when mass-production for washing, sorting, and packaging may spread bacterial contamination from a single egg to thousands being processed. Stay safe by following well-publicized guidelines for avoiding undercooked eggs. Never follow recipes where eggs are not thoroughly cooked unless you use pasteurized or irradiated eggs

The last agency that controls labeling is the Treasury Department. Because the government collects taxes on alcoholic beverages, Treasury decides the rules for alcoholic beverages. Beverages containing less than 0.5 percent of alcohol are considered non-alcoholic. This provision allows brewers to advertise beer as non-alcoholic, although it contains alcohol. This seems a small amount but can harm people who are attempting to avoid alcohol.

This problem does not apply to some newer, truly non-alcoholic beers, which say 0 percent alcohol on their label. Another problem for dieters is when the beer label provides a calorie count for carbohydrates. This seemingly helpful information is misleading since it ignores the calories that alcohol itself contains. Treat labels claims on alcoholic beverages as skeptically as anything else.

In today's complex world, knowing what goes into your body should be a right, not a privilege. Truthful and understandable labels have never harmed anyone.

Chapter 12:

Starting Out

Chapter 9 asked, "How can you find the right balance, a diet that can reverse insulin resistance and help you lose weight?" It described the characteristics of a diet that can do just that. They are:

- It should curb hunger, not cause hunger.
- It should use normal foods, not resort to exotic or expensive products.
- It should make smaller-portion sizes seem normal.
- It should allow enough variety so that you do not feel deprived.
- It should have a very low glycemic index and glycemic load.
- It should minimize your insulin needs, allowing your body to heal.
- It must be based upon solid physiologic principles, not wishful thinking.
- Its effectiveness should have been demonstrated for generations.

Chapter 12: Starting Out

I have been explaining, teaching and writing about such a diet for many years. I wrote a book about it,[48] *The New Hippocratic Diet,*® giving credit to Hippocrates, who used similar principles 2,400 years earlier. The principles of my diet have stood the test of time, as our underlying scientific knowledge of human physiology and biochemistry has grown. An expanded version of my book,[49] intended for people with Type II Diabetes, is called *Diabetes Recovery*. It contains additional information about the dietary control of diabetes.

This chapter explains how to start that diet, beginning with a few precautions. Chapters 5, 6 and 9 discussed whether you might need a professional's help in deciding whether you would benefit from dietary change. A few precautions are repeated here, as reminders. Some people should not do this alone; they should seek knowledgeable, professional care before starting. These include:

1. Anyone currently taking any form of diabetic medication.

2. Anyone taking medication affected by dietary choices and requiring blood tests, such as Lithium Carbonate or Warfarin.

3. Anyone who has had an eating disorder (such as bulimia) in the past or who expects to diet inconsistently.

---

48. Cohen, I. A., ***Dr. Cohen's New Hippocratic Diet**® **Guide: How to Really Lose Weight and Beat the Obesity Epidemic**.* Center for Health Information, 2008. ISBN 978-0-9820111-9-5.
• A Spanish-language version is also available.
Cohen, I. A. ***La Nueva Dieta Hipocrática: Cómo realmente bajar de peso y vencer las epidemias de obesidad y diabetes**.* Center for Health Information, 2013. ISBN 978-0-9820111-8-8.

49. Cohen, I.A. ***Diabetes Recovery: Reversing Diabetes with the New Hippocratic Diet**.*® Center for Health Information, 2010. ISBN 978-0-9820111-0-2

4. Anyone who is now pregnant or plans to become pregnant while dieting.

If any of these describe you, follow the matching numbered information below about precautions you will need to follow:

1. If you are taking any diabetic medication, you will have to plan with your doctor to reduce or stop that medication as soon as you start on the diet. All people taking diabetic medication should know that reducing their food intake, for any reason, will trigger a dangerous hypoglycemic episode unless they reduce medication. Your health professional should have explained this to you when you first started diabetic medication.

You should continue your home-glucose monitoring and discuss the results quickly and frequently with your doctor. The goal is the eventual elimination or reduction of these medications as your body recovers. Progress will vary, and your plan should be individualized, so work with your doctor. This is not a do-it-yourself project.

None of this applies to Type 1 diabetics. They must continue their use of insulin. Their situation is very different. This plan is not intended for Type 1 diabetics.

2. If you are taking a medicine that requires your doctor to use laboratory tests to check your blood level, you must work with your doctor. You do not want to change the effectiveness of a medication. Two medications are of particular concern. Lithium Carbonate absorption can be altered by diet. Your use of green leafy vegetables alters the effectiveness of the blood thinner Warfarin. There may be other suitable medications, or you may require extra monitoring. If

you use either of these medicines, work out an individualized plan with your physician.

3. If, in the past, you have had an eating disorder, such as bulimia, do not diet unless you are working with a knowledgeable and supportive professional. You may find this diet easy and effective when done correctly, but a professional's support will help prevent behavior that could harm you.

If you plan to combine features of different diets, think of the Danish proverb, "He who builds to every man's advice will have a crooked house." Once you commit, stick to it. Working a plan part-time or mixing features and ideas of differing diets will usually fail and might be dangerous.

Support groups that provide emotional support can help. These can be a group of friends informally helping each other at work, at your house of worship, or in a similar setting. Their focus should be support, not dietary advice or criticism, and definitely not any product sales. You might look into a self-help group such as Overeaters Anonymous.

Don't plan to start any ketogenic diet while you are pregnant. The best choice is to deal with weight loss and control of insulin resistance through diet first and plan to switch to a maintenance diet before pregnancy. Pregnancy in the animal kingdom is often over the winter, which combines pregnancy and ketosis. However, medical understanding is sparse about the safety of ketogenic dieting in pregnant women. Play it safe to protect your developing child.

Gestational diabetes, which shows up when you are

pregnant, has to be taken very seriously. Work closely with your obstetrician and consider following the type of a modified Mediterranean maintenance diet (discussed in Chapter 14) while pregnant.

Some women who had been infertile before dieting may suddenly find themselves pregnant, which happens because dieting reduces the insulin resistance underlying polycystic ovary syndrome. If you are trying to become pregnant, this diet may help you., and it is sometimes tried as a treatment for infertile women. However, if you are trying to avoid pregnancy and are sexually active, be sure you are practicing birth control.

Nursing mothers will find when they diet medical knowledge on macronutrient balance for their babies is sparse.[50] Because you are nursing, your baby will receive a diet high in the healthy butterfat of mother's milk. Research has shown that mothers' milk can contain between 6 percent and almost 30 percent butterfat, much higher than most formulas and commercial cows' milk! Babies who have been nursed are healthier and less likely to become obese as children.

Many women are interested in weight loss after childbirth, so many nursing mothers diet. We need better science showing how such dieting affects a mother's milk quality. For now, pay attention to your baby's satisfaction from nursing. Work with your baby's pediatrician to assure that your baby is growing and developing properly.

---

50. Golan, Y. et al. **Genetic and Physiological Factors Affecting Human Milk Production and Composition.** *Nutrients* 2020, *12*, 1500.

Chapter 12:   Starting Out

Beginning Your Diet

Pick a day when you are ready to start. It could be today or this weekend, but realize that the first day or two are the toughest. You are trying something new and may feel a bit irritable. That improves rapidly, but start your diet when you do not have to be pleasant to those around you! Don't try to ease your way into this diet or do it a little at a time. If you do, your brain will try to pull you back into your old habits. For the first few days, you may feel stressed. Psychological tricks will not work by themselves since your body is experiencing a physical change. If you do not accept that the struggle is real, you set yourself up for disappointment. Think of people who judge themselves and believe they are flawed as they struggle to give up addictive habits such as cigarette smoking.

Changing your eating pattern in an age where addictive food surrounds you can be just as tough as giving up an addictive drug. That is why you must do it quickly and forcefully. The founders of Alcoholics Anonymous, when describing their experiences quitting alcohol, used the phrase "half measures availed us nothing." That sentiment is equally applicable when you are changing your diet. Picture a person who sits on the fence, a picket fence with sharp points. You will be equally uncomfortable unless you tell your body you do not need sugar. You have a few days' worth of stored sugar energy (in the form of a starch called glycogen), which provides a steady supply of sugar for your brain and muscles.

When your blood sugar level falls, your brain responds with anxiety, a normal survival signal that drives hunger. Once your brain recognizes it is not going to get more sugar, it responds differently. At that point, your body begins to metabolize fat as its main energy source, and you become relaxed. Your body has entered ketosis, and your brain then increases its level of gamma-aminobutyric acid (GABA). That is a chemical that nature uses to calm you down. This has a purpose so that when you turn to your stored supply of fat energy, you are no longer bothered by the anxiety signal of a fluctuating sugar level.

Dieters not recognizing that natural mechanism is the reason so many diets fail. If you eat foods that flood you with unneeded sugar instead of following this natural pattern, that action snaps your brain back into a sugar craving. The secret of successful dieting is to avoid foods that create powerful signals to go back to old eating habits. Psychology alone can not override the biochemical and physiological responses that are hardwired into your system. You are a whole person, and you must respect the powerful nature of that balance.

The quickest and most effective way to initiate a diet is with a total fast. That can be done by temporarily avoiding any food that provides you energy. Non-calorie drinks are fine. If you desire to consume some food, you can modify that fast with small amounts of food with energy almost exclusively from fat. Examples are avocados, sour cream, real homemade whipped cream, and real cream in your coffee. Having the right foods on hand when you start is important. If you live by yourself, clearing out foods you do not want is equally important. Helpful suggestions and lists are in the Appendix at the back of this book.

We live in a sugar-crazed society, where you may not

Chapter 12: Starting Out

have used fat as your primary energy source since you were a nursing infant. Your body uses separate biochemical pathways to use energy in one form or another. The biochemical pathways needed to create ketosis and burn fat efficiently are there, waiting to be used, but are relatively weak from not having been well-used. Individual responses to starting will differ. Some people will convert into efficient fat burning within a day, but others might take several days, depending upon your past eating pattern. Once that change occurs, you will sense it rapidly. You will go from feeling hungry to not having the same powerful desire to eat.

There are ways of objectively measuring this change that you can use at home. Once your body begins to burn fat efficiently, your liver turns fat into ketones that your cells burn for energy. Ketosis means ketones are circulating in your blood, and ketogenic means a food mixture that supports ketosis. Measuring ketones give you a way to know how well you are doing objectively. There are three different ways to measure ketosis because three separate chemicals are created in ketosis. Any one can be measured at home, and which one you use may be based upon cost and convenience.

The least expensive and most common method of measuring ketosis is a urine test. When you are experiencing ketosis, the chemical **acetoacetic** acid will appear in your urine. You can buy a bottle with 50 test strips called **ketone test strips**[51] inexpensively at any pharmacy. You test your urine by holding the strip so that you dampen a little patch of chemically treated paper in your urine stream. The treated strip

---

51. Such as brand-name **Ketostix®**

should change color in about 15 seconds. You compare the color to a chart on the bottle to determine the amount of ketosis. At first, you may check more frequently, but once you are in ketosis, you should still check once or twice a day. The only drawback is that your urine does not reflect what is going on at that very instant. It shows what was going on in your blood over the past few hours. It may vary during the day, particularly if you exercise heavily and you burn off your ketones and there is little left to spill into your urine. Since the cost is only a few cents for each test, this is most common method. I recommend this, but some people also try two other methods.

The second method is less commonly used. It measures the chemical beta-hydroxybutyrate in a blood sample. This is the most abundant ketone and provides an accurate picture of what is going on at that moment. However, It requires purchasing a special meter, requires pricking your finger and costs about ten times as much for each test.

The newest method measures the chemical acetone on your breath. Specialized breath meters to detect acetone vary widely, from less than $50 to several hundred dollars. Their sensors are usable for a few hundred tests. The cheaper models are disposable, while the more expensive models may be sent back to the manufacturer to have the sensor replaced. Over time, the average cost per test may be reasonable, but the initial investment is a deterrent.

Before you reach ketosis, you are transitioning from sugar to fat for your energy. You may feel weaker, and your thinking might be a bit slower during the first day or two. Once

Chapter 12: Starting Out

you start ketosis, you will feel better. The calmness caused by ketosis should feel pleasant, and your energy and clarity should feel normal. Since you have not been using these biochemical pathways, they are weaker at first. You may not notice this in routine activities, but might feel exhausted if you work out strenuously. It may take a full month to reach your previous peak stamina level. If you exercise regularly, reduce your routine slightly and gradually build back up.

I recommend taking a daily fiber supplement and vitamin and mineral supplements from the very beginning. Which ones are right for you and the reasons for needing them are discussed in the Appendix.

Once you have succeeded in reaching ketosis, it is time to move on and begin to eat regularly, but staying within the new patterns that will help strengthen you and aid your resistance. Their purpose is not to starve you, but to teach you how to obtain, prepare, and enjoy real food that will let your body heal. Reverse your insulin resistance and its associated inflammation, reverse overweight, but enjoy the journey as you become healthier. Getting and staying healthy while at the same time protecting yourself from Covid-19 and other threats should be an enjoyable journey, not be a burden.

Chapter 13

Metabolism Improvement

Congratulations on reaching this point. Don't skip the initiation in the last chapter. Your success depends on working this program right, starting with that first initiation step. The earlier chapters provided background information. Now, you can implement what you learned. You are working on a lifetime plan for improving your metabolism, abolishing insulin resistance and restoring your immune response. Doing so strengthens your ability to fight off Covid-19 but goes much further in making you healthier. Achieving this goal is more than just trying a few recipes, it is a recipe for living. If you have gone through the initiation, congratulations again. Now, you are ready to move forward.

The instructions here are for a combined metabolism improvement and weight loss. Most people reading this will need to do both at first and then go on to that metabolism improvement. If you do not need to lose weight, spend a shorter time following the plan in this chapter, then move to the maintenance stage, explained in the next chapter. Either way, you'll find yourself on a new and enjoyable path.

An editor who assisted with this book disclosed that she

Chapter 13: Metabolism Improvement

started following it while editing this material and lost twenty-five pounds and was no longer in a pre-diabetic state. That is not unusual. A chiropractor, who was a student when her school invited me to lecture, called me several years later. She bought my book, followed it, and lost sixty pounds. After graduation, she was determined to carry this knowledge to her patients, and she has. A physician, attending a recent medical lecture I gave, took my online patient education course and lost seventy pounds. As he lost weight, his patients noticed and followed his example. What is special about these people (and many others) is that they were not my patients. They did not intentionally seek individual health or dietary advice. Instead, they learned of my program by chance, went on to read one of my books, or view my online course and gained the same knowledge that you are receiving from this book. That was enough to change their lives and inspire others.

During this initial stage, two things count: what you eat and how much you eat. To succeed, you need a balance between these to suppress your appetite. **The paradox is that eating a little more makes you hungrier.** When you are in ketosis, eating a little more may trick your body and your mind into believing you no longer are trying to burn off fat and cause you to regain sugar-driven cravings. That efficient fat-burning state is the process that makes you enjoy smaller quantities of real food yet feeling satisfied.

You may have heard that ketogenic diets allow you to ignore how much you eat, as long as you maintain a certain ratio between the types of food you eat. Sorry, but that only applies to strictly therapeutic ketogenic diets when no weight loss is attempted. They are discussed along with maintenance diets in the next chapter. If you have any expectation of losing weight, you must follow some simple guidelines for ketogenic weight-loss.

The good news is that a combined weight-loss and therapeutic ketogenic diet is **easier** to follow than a strictly therapeutic ketogenic diet. The proportion of fat to non-fat in the food you eat is not as extreme; your body will add to the fat you burn from your unwanted, stored fat. In a strictly therapeutic ketogenic diet, that is not the case, and you would have to eat a larger amount of fat in your diet. Some suggested daily menus in the Appendix, along with some recipes which will show you how easy following this diet is.

You will have to keep track of three forms of food energy. This is easier than it sounds if you follow the recipes given here or in our cookbook ***Cooking for the New Hippocratic Diet*®** (mentioned in Chapter 9), since those recipes provide the information you need. These three forms of energy are **fats, proteins** and **carbohydrates**. We discuss their amounts in grams, which is how they are shown in the Nutrition Facts box on product labels and recipes. Grams are not the same as the item's total weight. The total weight describes your serving size, but record the separate grams for each of these three macronutrients in your diary or other record.

Fats in your diet come from many sources. Your body can create certain types of fat on its own, but you must take in many fats to stay healthy. In addition to being used for energy, fats are structural elements in your body, especially your

Chapter 13: Metabolism Improvement

nervous system and are important components of hormones. The fats that you use but cannot produce yourself are called **essential fatty acids**. You cannot live on a diet totally devoid of fat. When fat is used for energy, one gram of fat produces nine calories of energy. One ounce is equal to about twenty-eight grams. Fat produces the greatest amount of energy for a given weight of any nutrient, making fat the ideal substance for your body to store the energy it needs for long-term use.

Proteins are essential building blocks for your body and are made up of **amino acids**. Your body constantly replaces worn-out cells with new ones. If you are in the process of healing, growing, or are pregnant, your body builds a greater number of cells. When you eat protein, your body breaks it into amino acids, which are reassembled into fresh new protein. Some of these amino acids can be made from scratch, but other amino acids must come from proteins that you eat. These are called **essential amino acids**. For that reason, you cannot live without some protein in your diet. During a famine in developing countries, children deprived of protein develop a disease known as *kwashiorkor* and will not survive without protein.

In developed countries, people generally eat an abundance of protein. When your body does not need this additional protein, it can be converted to energy, but cells of your body cannot burn protein directly. Instead, the amino acids enter the chemical pathways for either fat or sugar. The proportion going to either pathway depends on that particular protein's amino acid composition, but it is roughly a 50/50 split. People with diabetes who monitor their blood sugar will notice that it rises after a large protein meal. The extra chemical steps needed to turn protein into energy make that blood sugar rise gradual, but it is still present.

Carbohydrates represent the most common energy source, yet they can be the most dangerous when eaten in excess. You need to maintain a blood-sugar level for certain functions, even when your body is in ketosis. Carbohydrates are made up of sugars and starches, most of which get turned into glucose or blood sugar. When there is more sugar than you need at the moment, insulin signals your liver to convert that sugar to fat and then send that fat into storage. Your body can function without ever eating carbohydrates because **there are no essential carbohydrates.**

Fiber is also a carbohydrate chemically, but it has no nutritive value as energy in humans. When dieting or otherwise counting your energy input, don't count the fiber! Since the government counts fiber as a carbohydrate in the nutrition label, remember to subtract it from the total carbohydrate count. The resulting number is popularly called ***net carbs.*** The recipes in this book provide a net carb amount when listing carbohydrate content.

Grazing animals break the fiber cellulose in the grass that they eat and absorb the energy from it—part of the cycle of nature. The sun's energy is captured in growing grass and grazing animals take in that energy. Humans or other animals, in turn, eventually benefit from those grazing animals. The fiber in human diets is beneficial, but not for energy. Fiber from green leafy vegetables and other sources helps add bulk to your waste, keeping your digestive system healthy.

Chapter 13: Metabolism Improvement

When a patient is interested in losing weight and maintaining a state of ketosis at the same, I often recommend a daily allowance of:

60 grams of fat,
40 grams of protein and
10 grams of carbohydrates.

This recommendation is not universal. As I explained earlier, some people should not diet or should receive individual direction from their physician. However, this **60-40-10** mixture works well with most people. I developed it from the Total Ketogenic Ratio calculations using the algorithm explained in Chapter 9 and have presented this information at many scientific medical forums over the years. The best way to describe this diet is *moderate fat, moderate protein, and very low carbohydrate.* Full-energy ketogenic diets usually need to be high in fat to maintain ketosis. However, when weight reduction is involved, they must take into account the stored fat burned. That reduces the need to eat higher fat levels since **60 grams of fat** is less than the total fat in the American Heart Association's "Low-Fat" standard diet, although it may seem proportionately high compared to other things that you eat. Should you eat additional fat, you would stay in ketosis, but it will slow your weight loss.

Forty grams of protein is a lot less than you may be used to but is more than adequate for most adults who do not have special protein needs. People who need more protein might be healing from an accident or surgery, engaged in heavy physical activity, still growing, or pregnant. If any of these apply to you, your physician may suggest a different protein amount. Keep in mind that too much protein will be turned into energy and can increase your blood sugar.

Finally, you can allow yourself **up to 10 grams of carbohydrate** each day. You do not need any carbohydrates in your diet, but this is an allowance so that you may eat foods that contain small amounts of carbohydrates. As an example, eating green leafy vegetables is encouraged. Since you are using "net carbs," you will find that the amount of carbohydrates in many green leafy vegetables is small once you deduct the fiber.

This **60-40-10** formula works for most people. Physically small adults who are overweight may require some slight downward adjustment. People who are significantly obese will still do well on this small amount, without adjustment. On average, a loss of two pounds per week is a good target for many people. In the first few days of initiation, many people will lose more, but they will settle down to a steady weekly loss in the long run. **60-40-10** represents actual grams in each category every day. <u>It is not a ratio or a percentage</u>, but the actual amount of each nutrient daily. Use the nutritional analysis for each food to determine how many grams of each category it contains.

Paying attention to exactly what you have eaten on any day may seem tedious, but it is worthwhile. An example of a daily diary can be found at the end of this chapter. Readers can freely copy it for their personal use. A diary is worthwhile since it teaches you how food is affecting you. Keeping this record allows you to see what works and what does not work. It is best to keep your diary in your pocket or purse to use it when

Chapter 13: Metabolism Improvement

you eat. It is more difficult to correctly remember everything you have done if you wait until the end of the day to record it.

Some people prefer to use apps on their phones, and others create spreadsheets. If you use either of those, use the format in the sample diary. It contains information you will find helpful. For example, if your morning weight shows a loss of 4 ounces or one-quarter of a pound every day, it seems like a small amount to keep track of, yet it amounts to one and three-quarter pounds each week. Over six months, you should lose more than forty-five pounds. If you were doing that on a steady basis and then noticed a few days where you lost nothing or even gained a few ounces, your diary gives you the ability to check and discover why. Your diary is an important teaching tool. It puts you in control, letting you learn how your body works.

If this sounds like a lot of work, remember why you are doing this. Your weight is a marker, telling you a lot about your metabolism and health. These steps you're taking can bring you back to better health and will do so long before you reach any target weight. Inflammation from insulin resistance does damage itself while also making you more susceptible to severe consequences, should you become infected. Long after this epidemic ends, the benefits of what you're doing today will continue to help you.

Where will the numbers for your diary come from? If you start with the recipes in this book and our cookbook, you will find the numbers right there. If you buy processed food with a label, use the numbers from that label. If you purchase fresh produce or meats and poultry, there are ways to look it up. One way is to purchase a book called a **complete food counter**. These handy books are inexpensive and available through bookstores or the internet. Be sure to look for one that is **complete** since many food-counting books just list partial information tied to various fad diets. A complete food counter should show you the amount of fat, protein, and carbohydrates in a particular food item. Ignore the many pages of products with labels since the labeled product in your hands is the latest one. Use the book for the contents of fresh food that does not have any label. If you don't have such a book at hand, the internet may provide you answers. Use the words "Nutritional Analysis" and the name of the food, and you are likely to find a few sites that provide that information.

When you are in ketosis, you may find yourself satisfied even while skipping meals. People are conditioned to believe in three fixed meals a day, a cultural standard that varies worldwide. When you are eating high carbohydrate foods, rising and falling blood sugar requires you to eat more frequently. School programs that feed children breakfast so they will be focused enough to learn are a consequence of poor home nutrition problems. The need for a mid-morning coffee break is another consequence of rising and falling blood sugar.

When you are in ketosis, your body has a steady supply of fat for energy, and your blood sugar is relatively constant. As a result, many people are not hungry for their routine three meals. If this happens to you, it is okay to make adjustments. You might only want two meals a day or even just one. Listen to your body. Pay attention to whether you are fatigued or have

Chapter 13: Metabolism Improvement

good energy and are clearheaded. Make your own decisions about what is right for you.

As you progress, note the changes. Accept that you have made progress and deserve credit for what you've done. Those around you may not compliment you readily. People are sensitive about their weight, so others may be reluctant to say something at first. Friends and relatives who you have not seen for a long time are more likely to speak up than those close to you who gradually see changes. If you feel good, it is okay to mention it to others.

People around you may be skeptical when you start to lose weight, but you may become a leader once they see you succeed. People often form casual support groups, a few friends or coworkers following the same plan provide someone to talk to and share ideas with. Knowing that other people are succeeding in the same way you are can be a big boost when you have questions or face a rough day. Some people might benefit from a support group such as Overeaters Anonymous. They will not provide you dietary advice but may help with self-esteem issues that can undermine your recovery process. If you have a personal physician, improvements in your physical status may be reinforced by progress in objective laboratory tests. These can add to the feeling you have accomplished something useful. Stick to your plan, get those results to improve and feel better! Don't be afraid to use personal goals that others might not understand. Just being able to play with your children or grandchildren once again can be reinforcement enough.

On the next page there is a diary to copy for your

Fighting Covid-19, the Unequal Opportunity Killer

Date:			This is day	of my diet.		
New Hippocratic Diet ® Daily Diary							
Time	Food Item, Test or Weight	Test Results	FAT grams 60 x9	PROTEIN grams 40 x4	CARBS grams 10 x4	calories (optional)
	Daily Totals	add columns	grams	grams	grams	calories
Special events and comments						

© Irving A. Cohen
all rights reserved

personal use or download it from www.HippocraticDiet.com. A sample follows, showing a completed page with instructions illustrating how to use it. Next, Chapter 14 will teach you how to stay metabolically safe and healthy once you reach your weight

Chapter 13: Metabolism Improvement

Date: July 1   **This is day** 38 **of my diet.**

New Hippocratic Diet™ Daily Diary

Time	Food Item or Test or Weight	Test Results	FAT grams 60 x9	PROTEIN grams 40 x4	CARBS grams 10 x4	calories (optional)
6:30	weight	237 1/2				
"	glucose	97				
"	ketosis	large				
7:15	Coffee + tbs. cream		5	-	-	
"	omelet		11 (44)	6 (36)	1 (9)	
9:15	glucose	108				
10:30	Coffee + tbs. cream		5	-	-	
12:45	Salad, blue cheese		6	2	4	
"	Cream soda		5 (28)	- (34)	- (5)	
2:45	glucose	109				
6 pm	ketosis	moderate				
"	weight	238				
6:30	3 oz salmon/oil		11	20	-	
"	4 Asparagus		-	1	2	
"	Curry sauce		11	-	-	
"	Iced tea		- (6)	- (13)	- (3)	
8:30	glucose	110				
9 pm	Munster cheese x2		10	12	-	
		Daily Totals add columns	64 (576) grams	39 (156) grams	7 (28) grams	780 calories

Special events and comments

Felt great during the day, had a high energy level.
Had 2 slices of cheese as a snack at night.

Fighting Covid-19, the Unequal Opportunity Killer

loss goal.

Track your progress by using a daily diary page. Write the numbers in from every item you eat so that by the end of the day, you can see how close you are to your **60-40-10** goal.

Some people prefer to subtract each item's value from **60-40-10** as the day goes on, noting how much remains at a glance. It is not necessary to record calories. They are there for people who prefer to list them. If you do, the numbers 9, 4, and 4 at the top of the gram columns are there as a reminder. Multiply fat grams by 9, protein grams by 4, and carbohydrate grams by 4 to determine calories.

Use the "Results" column to track your glucose readings (if you use these), ketosis tests, and your weight. If you fill these out regularly, you will see how closely you are following the diet, what foods have an impact, and keep you in ketosis. As a result, you will see what eating patterns help you lose weight. Remember to compare morning weights to each other, not to evening weights, which will differ. Use the time column to show the time of test readings and meals.

The completed sample page shows how one woman used her diary:

- She entered the date and day of dieting for future reference.
- She started the day recording her weight and test results.
- After meals, she subtracted her grams from the **60-40-10** reminders at the top of the columns to see how much she had left to work with during the day.

Chapter 13: Metabolism Improvement

- Her urine test for ketosis was large in the morning but slightly less during the active day when her body was burning ketones as fast as it was creating them.

- Her weight went up slightly during the day, which is normal, and the following morning it should be less than this morning.

- At the end of the day, she totaled up 64-39-7, close to her goal of **60-40-10**. She was curious about calories, so at the end of the day, she used the numbers at the top of the columns (9-4-4) to multiply the gram totals and calculate her total calories.

As you watch your progress and your weight continues to fall, your diary will provide a reminder of what you have done so far and a tool to teach you how to do your best. Keep your diary. The information you will be learning about yourself will help you again when you are maintaining healthy metabolism in the future.

Chapter 14

One Day at a Time

The last thirteen chapters have guided you in becoming healthier. Now, it's time to stay healthier, one day at a time. We live in a culture obsessed with selling products that supposedly will make you healthier, or at least that's what they claim. Whether it's the television networks or social media you follow, these champions of good health always have something to sell. There are magic pills to make you young again, food subscription plans, sugar-laden breakfast cereals, and smartwatches all claiming to be good for your health.

The truth is, most of them do not work. By following this diet, you have crafted your own path to better health, and now you want to stay on that path. If you were overweight and slimmed-down, if you had diabetes and no longer need medication, if you have reversed insulin-resistance inflammation, you have accomplished major changes in your health. Perhaps you were exposed to Covid-19 but only developed a few mild symptoms. These are real changes, and you should be proud of what you have accomplished.

The question is, what to do next? Maintaining your improvement requires two things. First, you need to know

Chapter 14:   One day at a time

where you are. You may have lost a huge amount of weight and feel that that is enough in itself. That may be, but has your body had enough time to reverse all of the insulin resistance you were dealing with? Objective tests described in Chapter 6 are good markers. If they have reached healthy values, you have accomplished quite a bit. If they are better but still not ideal, you want to remain vigilant.

Either way, you want to avoid the yo-yo effect that comes with so many fads, commercial diets, and diet drug use. You have learned what is good and bad in the foods you eat. Now, you can use that knowledge to develop your maintenance plan. If you kept a food diary, refer to it now. It can serve as your reminder of what worked well and what did not.

Another important factor is knowledge of what your ancestors' diet was when they were free and prosperous. This may be impossible for some of us since history may have erased large blocks of information. What we might think of as traditional food reflects what your family ate during times of deprivation. Try to find how they ate during the good times if there were any, which may give you connectedness to your ancient roots and strengthen your resolve to eat healthily.

When Spanish forces enslaved Native Americans, they deprived them of their usual varied diet and their health deteriorated rapidly. When the Army forced removal of Native Americans westward on the Trail of Tears, rations were limited to lard and flour, which resulted in the invention of fry bread. Today, fry bread is celebrated as a traditional food; yet, it represents an unhealthy legacy of deprivation. The British conquest of Ireland forced many people to subsist on potatoes grown in their gardens, while the pasturelands produced beef and butter for export to Britain. When the potato crop failed, millions starved yet landowners exported healthy food. Similar events occurred for many groups and in many times. If you can discover things about your ancestors' diet during good times, it can strengthen your belief in healthy traditional foods for a maintenance diet.

Discover the seasonality and variety of local foods. Shop at farmers' markets. Look into fresh foods that might be available in your locale by visiting www.localharvest.com.

Make the transition to your maintenance lifestyle gradual, one day at a time. If you transition to a diet that is no longer ketogenic, expect to see a small weight increase in the first few days. When you started, your weight rapidly dropped as you used your stored sugar supply. That quick loss of a few pounds of weight was not fat burning, so when you leave ketosis, your body will rebuild that stored supply of sugar. Gaining a few pounds in the first few days is normal and does not mean you are putting fat back on.

Continue to limit yourself to very little sugar and few carbohydrate-rich foods. Use moderation in choosing the amount of protein you plan to eat. Continue to include fat in your diet, favoring healthy natural fats and avoiding human-made and chemically engineered fats. Pay attention to the ingredients in your food, and continue to avoid the appetite-increasing flavor enhancer chemicals. Prefer truly natural foods, but be wary of food manufacturers' misuse of the word "natural."

Whatever maintenance diet choice you take, make the

Chapter 14: One day at a time

transition gradually. If you feel better when on the diet, you don't want to lose that good feeling. This usually happens from several causes working together. Ketosis itself can make you feel good because it changes your brain chemistry. You might have also felt good because you were no longer eating a particular item you were sensitive to. It may have been a flavor-enhancing chemical. It may have been a natural substance, such as gluten found in grain products. For all these reasons, transition a day at a time. Treat everything you add or go back to like something new and take on each new item separately. Take a few days to see if a new item has negative effects. Some might be trigger foods, ones that may make you want to overeat. This can happen because that particular food manipulates your blood sugar level or because it evokes memories attached to that food. Either way, it may be a pitfall for you.

You have choices about types of maintenance diet to follow, but they all overlap. At one extreme, you could go back to eating "regular" foods, but maintain a low glycemic-index diet and watch the portion size. The danger here would be in overconfidence, believing you have done so well that you allow yourself to backslide.

At the other extreme, you can continue in ketosis but increase your food intake so that you are no longer losing weight. This might be the right choice if ketosis itself seems very comfortable for you. It requires you to increase the amount of fat in your diet since you will no longer be burning your stored body fat. In this case, your maintenance diet will become a therapeutic ketogenic diet. Typically, that can mean you have to maintain three or four times as much fat (in grams) as non-fat (protein plus carbohydrate). In other words, olive oil and butter become your best friends. Most people do not have to go this far, but if you find yourself agitated or if your blood sugar level is bouncing like a yo-yo, it is worth considering.

Although ketosis itself brought about increases in brain GABA, creating a calm mental state, you might investigate other things you can also do to create a calm and satisfied feeling. For some people, meditation, exercise, yoga, or a tai chi program might help bring the clarity and calmness they found while dieting. Others can find inner calmness in a hobby such as woodworking, painting, knitting, or hiking.

In between these two extremes, a healthy and pleasant option is what I call a "Modified Mediterranean-Style Diet." The popularized "Mediterranean Diet" is not exactly what I mean. Much had been claimed about the health benefits of the so-called Mediterranean Diet in recent years, but in truth, the diets of nations bordering the Mediterranean Sea vary widely. Some poorer Mediterranean regions rely heavily on inexpensive grains. Although olive oil is synonymous with a truly healthy Mediterranean diet, the average consumption of olive oil can vary by a factor of ten or twenty times between different parts of the Mediterranean. Geography, agricultural practices, and culture mean that the Mediterranean has many different diets. The people of Greece use healthy olive oil at many times the rate of their neighbors and produce more high-quality olive oil than any other place on earth. In addition, in the past, the Greek Isles' different topography meant that their diet was healthier than that of the Greek mainland. That is the type of

Chapter 14: One day at a time

diet I recommend.

The wonderful diet of that region is a result of Greek geography. The mainland of Greece allows various crops, but the Greek Isles' rugged terrain made the olive tree a preferred agricultural crop and a major food source. In ancient times, the olive became a source of wealth as the Greeks exported this healthy oil throughout the ancient world. Today, the average consumption of olive oil per person in Greece is more than twenty times that of the average American. Looking at domestic use of olive oil, the average Greek may consume almost a third of their energy intake from this healthy food. Importantly, the Mediterranean Sea surrounding the Greek Isles provides a wealth of fresh fish that is another integral part of that Greek eating tradition.

In addition to the fat coming from olive oil, Greeks consume other fats from fish, nuts, meat, cheese and other dairy products. The total of all those fats can be well above the 30 percent energy recommendation from fat that heart experts talk about in the United States. Yet Greeks have a lower level of heart disease than we do here in America. The positive benefit of a diet high in such healthy and natural fats is found in Greece.

Protein from fish, meat, and eggs are present in moderate amounts, but what about carbohydrates? Today, bread plays a role in Greek diets but transporting grain from the mainland before steam power made this costlier in the isles. The rugged topography made grain difficult to grow in the islands, although olive trees and vegetable gardens fared well. With a higher proportion of healthy fat, fewer calories from other sources, such as carbohydrates, were needed to fulfill people's energy needs.

Find your comfort zone in choosing your style of maintenance dieting. When you chose to include some carbohydrates, mixtures of vegetables, including peas and beans with only limited whole grain, are the healthiest carbohydrate mixture. However, if you have found that you were previously addicted to carbohydrates, be cautious, for even moderate amounts of these might be triggers to overconsumption.

Don't deny yourself all pleasures. Instead, treat special things with the appreciation that comes from their rarity. Savoring very modest amounts of fresh fruit as it comes into the season is an example of allowing yourself only modest amounts of high sugar foods, yet appreciating these occasional gifts. Using the seasonality of local items will make you appreciate them more. Items such as festive pastries covered with honey should be restricted to rare holidays and family occasions. Even then, if you have diabetes, monitor your blood glucose carefully to tell you what, how much, and how often you can tolerate these as additions to your diet. Never consider yourself cured of those dietary mistakes that harmed you in the past. Instead, think of yourself as someone in remission from that harmful past. **Let those mistakes stay in your past.**

High carbohydrate food had its place in human history, so you do not have to demonize it. As human civilization grew, changing agricultural techniques allowed more people to be fed. In many places, social stratification grew along with population. Often, the lowest ranks had limited diets while the

Chapter 14: One day at a time

upper classes "lived off the fat of the land." Historically, the poorest people may have had just enough food to get by. Their very poverty might have protected them from the dangers of overconsumption if they didn't die of starvation. Diseases associated with dietary overindulgence were more likely to be found among the rich or powerful. Today, food production advances allow both rich and poor to overindulge. The paradox is that many people eat poorly, believing they are eating healthily. Manufacturers continue to find new ways to substitute imitations made from inexpensive ingredients and try to convince people they are improvements. Please, don't fall for it.

When the Second World War ended, food in Europe was scarce, but surprisingly death rates fell, despite the deprivation. Massive humanitarian U.S. food aid as well as the rebuilding of infrastructure restored Europe's food supply, and death rates once again climbed. Feeding people what was considered enough food brought on higher death rates. Both historic epidemiology studies and animal experiments have repeatedly shown that limited energy in your diet makes your body more efficient and lengthens a healthy life.

Efforts to feed the world by simply increasing calories can have a deadly impact. Over a century of mass-produced, processed food has worsened this problem. The massive reliance on both sugar and flavor enhancers in such food products promotes overeating. Even our school systems threaten our children because they are burdened by regulations favoring mass-produced foods from the distant factories over healthier local foods.

Fighting Covid-19, the Unequal Opportunity Killer

Outdated assumptions continue to underlie many recommendations about nutrition. In trying to overcome malnutrition from the 1930s depression, the pendulum swung in the opposite direction. The middle of the 20th century saw a tremendous change in how people lived and the energy they need for routine tasks; yet, standards and programs are based upon needs that no longer exist. Many sedentary people do not require the standard recommended 2,000 or more calories each day. The number of calories that many people require today for a sedentary lifestyle may be as little as half of what was considered correct earlier in the 20th-century. The higher requirements for active lifestyles have changed even more. A "lumberjack's breakfast" with a huge stack of pancakes only worked when a lumberjack relied on an ax and bucksaw and burned 9,000 calories in a day's work. Rely on your own experience to learn what your needs are.

The point here is that quantity and purity both matter. Know what you're eating and how much you are eating to avoid returning to your previously unhealthy state. Pay attention to previous generations' wisdom, whether from Hippocrates, the Bible, or Benjamin Franklin. They all recommended moderation, although Mr. Franklin did not always follow his own advice. Know what is a moderate amount of food for you and what may drive you to overeat. Find comfort in the quality, not the quantity, of the food that you eat.

We do not know what the future will bring in terms of the end of this epidemic or the recurrence of waves of modified threats. We know that each of us has natural defenses, but

Chapter 14: One day at a time

these defenses are not absolute. Despite historic social, economic, or racial disparities that previously weakened your defenses, you can prevent them from pushing you back into a high-risk group. **You, not age nor privilege, should control your own body's ability to maintain its strong defenses.**

The purpose of this book has been twofold. First, to move you out of the high-risk category should you become infected by Covid-19. Second, to provide better health for you in the future.

Just remember that nothing here makes you bulletproof! Continue to take the guidelines regarding the routine use of masks and social distances very seriously. Research has demonstrated that these are effective tools in reducing exposure risk. If you have not already done so, get your flu vaccination. Early on, we heard predictions that the Covid-19 epidemic would worsen during the flu season. The good news is that worldwide surveillance shows there may not be a severe flu season in many parts of the world. Travel restrictions, flu vaccinations, and mask use have restricted flu dramatically.

Scientists, drug companies and governments around the world have worked remarkably hard to develop and produce effective and safe vaccines to protect against Covid-19. Accept vaccination as soon as it is available to you. Do not avoid vaccines by trying to rely on herd immunity to protect you. Herd immunity only works after many others have been infected or vaccinated. In the meantime, more people can become ill or die. In an epidemic, we must protect ourselves; yet, we must consider our surrounding community

Fighting Covid-19, the Unequal Opportunity Killer
simultaneously.

Following this chapter is an Appendix with much detailed information and many useful suggestions. It should answer many of the questions you have been asking as you read this book. Finally, I would like to provide you my best wishes in many languages;

To Health

pour la santé

do zdrowia

para la salud

für die Gesundheit

alla salute

para a saúde

לבריאות lechaim

بالصحة bialsiha

"The health of the people is really the foundation upon which all their happiness and all their powers as a state depend."

Benjamin Disraeli. 1877
Former British Prime Minister

Appendix

The purpose of this Appendix is to provide you with extra information and answer questions about diet such as: What should I eat? Should I take supplements? What ingredients are good for me? It is not intended to replace our other books, which you will find helpful and detailed.

Dealing with Dietary Restrictions

If you are already living with dietary restrictions, in most cases you can still follow the dietary guidelines simply by making adjustments to which recipes you select. This is a short discussion of what you may encounter or may have to modify. People follow dietary restrictions for a variety of reasons: medically imposed, religious observance, moral considerations and health beliefs.

Fat restrictions. Low carbohydrate ketogenic diets are often inaccurately described as high in fat. This is a half-truth. It is true for a therapeutic ketogenic diet, which must be high in fat, both proportionally and totally to achieve a ketogenic fat-burning state. That may have not be best for someone who has a valid medical restriction on fat. On the other hand, a properly designed ketogenic weight-loss diet, as described here, actually has **less total dietary fat** then a standard American Heart Association" low-fat" diet, despite having a higher proportion of dietary fat. This seeming contradiction is because the fat being burned from stored fat can be enough to maintain ketosis.

Salt restrictions. Salt restriction is a misnomer, because the actual restriction is a **sodium restriction.** By avoiding processed food that contains **monosodium glutamate,** whether hidden or labeled, you are already avoided the major source of sodium in the American diet.

Gluten-free. If you are avoiding gluten, this diet is perfect for you. All the recipes we use, both here and in our cookbook are gluten-free. This is

Appendix

actually better than typical gluten-free diets and gluten-free products, which may be loaded with rice flour and can increase your chances for weight gain and diabetes. Use caution in the marketplace, since there are a handful of products, such as "keto-friendly bread" which do not contain wheat but may contain extracted wheat gluten.

Jewish dietary traditions and Islamic dietary traditions. Either tradition can be followed easily by avoiding certain recipes or substituting certain ingredients.

Vegetarianism. Lacto-ovo vegetarians who will not eat animals but will consume dairy and eggs produced by animals have good sources of healthy fat and protein. As usual, for any form of vegetarianism, they may need a Vitamin B_{12} supplement.

Vegans are vegetarians who will not eat any product produced by animals such as dairy and eggs. They are one group that will have extreme difficulty finding acceptable dietary choices for following a true low carbohydrate diet while attempting to get enough protein from plant sources.

Meal Plans

When you begin your new diet, try to plan what to eat for the entire day. Your may be skeptical about the portion size but once you begin, you will be surprised at how satisfied you are. Since we are used to eating three meals a day, these sample meal plans include breakfast, lunch, and dinner. However, as your body moves away from the ups and downs of a high-carbohydrate lifestyle, you may find that you prefer to eat less often. Some people find they are comfortable with two meals a day or even just one! Whatever you choose to do, try to hit the target of 60 grams fat, 40 grams protein, and 10 grams or less carbohydrate. These meal plans roughly follow that guideline, but you should verify that these meet your needs. Feel free to adjust and switch these around, they are here for you only as a starting point.

Fighting Covid-19, the Unequal Opportunity Killer

Monday

Breakfast	Coffee with real cream and non-calorie sweetener
	One fluffy egg omelet *(see recipe #1)*
	One thick *(or 2 regular)* strip(s) sugar-free bacon *(if available)*
Lunch	Small lettuce salad with two grape tomatoes
	Shredded cheese
	Olive oil dressing
	Water or diet soda
Dinner	Three-to-four ounce steak
	Broccoli with melted cheese
	Water or diet soda
Optional snack	One-half ounce cashews

Tuesday

Breakfast	Coffee with real cream and non-calorie sweetener
	One fried egg
	One MSG-free sausage patty
Lunch	Small lettuce salad with two grape tomatoes
	Sliced cooked chicken *(about an ounce)*
	Bleu cheese dressing *(see recipe #2)*
	Water or diet soda
Dinner	Three to four ounce salmon portion
	Small lettuce salad with two grape tomatoes, shredded cheese and olive oil dressing
	Water or diet soda
Optional snack	One ounce of cheese cubes

Appendix

Wednesday

Breakfast	Homemade hot chocolate *(see recipe #3)*
	One scrambled egg
	One MSG-free sausage link
Lunch	MSG-free tuna salad on a bed of lettuce
	"Free lemonade" *(see recipe #4)*, water, or diet soda
Dinner	Four ounce pork chop with homemade barbecue sauce *(see recipe #5)*
	Small lettuce salad with two grape tomatoes, shredded cheese, and bleu cheese dressing *(see recipe #2)*
	Water or diet soda
Optional snack	One-half ounce almonds

Thursday

Breakfast	Coffee with real cream and non-calorie sweetener
	One scrambled egg mixed with one ounce cooked or smoked salmon
Lunch	Small portion mixed greens topped with smoked kippers
	Olive oil dressing
	Water or diet soda
Dinner	Chicken with Creamy Mustard Sauce *(see recipe #6)*
	Small lettuce salad with two grape tomatoes, shredded cheese, and olive oil dressing
	Water or diet soda
Optional snack	One ounce olives

Fighting Covid-19, the Unequal Opportunity Killer

Friday

Breakfast	Coffee with real cream and non-calorie sweetener
	One fluffy egg omelet *(see recipe)*
	One thick or 2 regular) strip*(s)* bacon *(sugar-free if available)*
Lunch	Small lettuce salad with two grape tomatoes
	Sliced cooked chicken *(about an ounce)*
	Bleu cheese dressing *(see recipe #2)*
	Water or diet soda
Dinner	Three-to-four ounces chicken topped with homemade mole sauce *(see recipe #9)*
	Small lettuce salad with and olive oil dressing
	Water or diet soda
Optional snack	Sugar-free Jell-O™ topped with homemade whipped cream *(see recipe #7)*

Saturday

Breakfast	Coffee with real cream and non-calorie sweetener
	One scrambled egg
	One thick or 2 regular) strip*(s)* bacon *(sugar-free if available)*
Lunch	Small lettuce salad with two grape tomatoes
	Sliced cooked chicken *(about an ounce)*
	Bleu cheese dressing *(see recipe #2)*
	Water or diet soda
Dinner	Four ounce portion lamb breast
	Lightly steamed asparagus with creamy curry sauce *(see recipe #10)*
	Water or diet soda
Optional snack	Real cream soda *(see recipe #8)*

Appendix

	Sunday
Breakfast	Coffee with real cream and non-calorie sweetener
	One fluffy egg omelet *(see recipe #1)*
	One MSG-free sausage link
Lunch	Small lettuce salad topped with sesame oil
	Chicken with Creamy Mustard Sauce *(see recipe # 6)*
	Water or diet soda
Dinner	Three-to-four ounce portion of salmon
	Small lettuce salad with two grape tomatoes, shredded cheese, and feta cheese dressing *(see recipe #2)*
	Water or diet soda
Optional snack	One ounce olives

Starter Recipes

The meal plans referred to a few special recipes that have been enjoyed by people who have used this diet. Each recipe includes its estimated energy content in grams and calories. Recipes containing fiber are adjusted to show only the value of the net carbohydrates. A much wider variety of recipes is found in our cookbook ***Cooking for the New Hippocratic Diet®*** ISBN 978-0-9820111-7-1 available at your favorite bookseller or from **www.EpidemicWall.com** .

Fighting Covid-19, the Unequal Opportunity Killer

1. Fluffy Egg Omelet

Nutritionally, this is the same as an omelet made in the normal way but once you try it, you will appreciate its flavor, texture, and size. Using a single egg, it provides about the same size portion as an ordinary two egg omelet. If you are not used to separating eggs, buy a simple egg separator at a kitchen or houseware store.

Ingredients	Amount
Large egg	1
Heavy cream	1 teaspoon
Extra-virgin olive oil (or butter)	1 teaspoon
Salt, pepper, or spice	to taste

Instructions: Separate the egg white from the yolk. Using an electric mixer or a hand whisk, beat the egg white until it is very frothy and increased in volume. Heat the olive oil (or butter) in a frying pan. Lightly blend the egg yolk and spices into the frothy egg white. Pour the mixture into the heated frying pan. Cook until done, flipping or covering to be sure that the top is done.

If you are cooking for several people, be sure to use a large pan. This recipe produces a thick, fluffy omelet. The air you whisked in will insulate the top of the omelet from the cooking heat unless you use a large pan to allow the mixture to spread out.

Energy	127 calories
Fat	11 grams
Protein	6 grams
Carbohydrate	1 gram

---

2. Chunky Bleu or Feta Cheese Dressing

Use this as a salad dressing, a sauce to top meat, fish and vegetables or as a dip for celery.

Ingredients	Amount
Crumpled bleu cheese or feta cheese	¼ cup
Real mayonnaise	½ cup
Real sour cream	1 cup
Hot sauce (optional)	a few drops, to taste
Salt, pepper, or spice	to taste

Instructions: Mix ingredients. Refrigerate unused portion.

Serving Size: About 2 tablespoons

Energy	62 calories
Fat	6 grams
Protein	6 grams
Carbohydrate	1 gram

Appendix

3. Hot Chocolate

Use this recipe when you need a chocolate lift or to warm yourself on a dreary winter day. You also may refrigerate it to serve cold, either by itself or mixed with club soda.

Ingredients	Amount
100% cocoa powder ¼ cup	1 teaspoon
Heavy cream	½ cup
Real sour cream	1 tablespoon
Non-calorie sweetener	to taste
Hot water	to fill cup

Instructions: Pour hot to boiling water over cocoa powder and stir until dissolved. Add cream, sweeten to taste and stir.

Energy	65 calories
Fat	5½ grams
Protein	1 gram
Carbohydrate	3 grams

---

4. Free Lemonade

This is a strategy to cope with problems when eating out, but it also works at home. When eating out, the only non-calorie beverage choices are often either water or something containing caffeine. If you do not want to have caffeine with your meal, too bad. Here is a way to fight back. It is free of both sugar and caffeine, as well as free-of-charge.

Ingredients	Amount
Water	1 glass
Lemon	1 slice
Non-calorie sweetener	to taste

Instructions: Ask your server for a slice of lemon in your water. Squeeze the lemon into you glass and use non-calorie sweetener to taste. Tip the staff a little more for their trouble, since you saved money compared to a soft drink. At home, you may use concentrated lemon or lime juice.

Energy   NONE

Fighting Covid-19, the Unequal Opportunity Killer

5. Barbecue and Meat Sauce

This is a terrific sauce for cooking meat and as a base for other sauces. It is calorie-free and can be made up in advance and stored. The key ingredient is a Mexican chipotle sauce, a thick brown sauce made from smoked chili peppers. Bufalo™ brand can be found in the Mexican food section of many supermarkets and specialty stores.

Ingredients	Amount
Chipotle sauce *(additive-free)*	All quantities to taste
Ground cinnamon	All quantities to taste
Non-calorie liquid sweetener	All quantities to taste
Fresh or bottled lemon juice	All quantities to taste

Instructions: Mix ingredients together until completely blended. Quantities can be varied to your taste. Brush on meat or chicken before cooking.

Energy   NONE

---

6. Chicken with Creamy Mustard Sauce

This is a tasty pan-fried dish.

Ingredients	Amount
Prepared mustard	½ teaspoon
Mayonnaise	½ teaspoon
Lime juice	¼ teaspoon
Olive oil	¼ teaspoon
Chicken leg	1

Instructions: Combine mustard, mayonnaise, and lime juice, and stir well. Heat oil in a frying pan and add chicken. Cover and cook 12 to 15 minutes until chicken is cooked, using medium heat and turning once. Remove chicken and place on a serving platter. Add mustard mixture to pan drippings and stir. Spoon mixture over chicken and serve.

Energy	375 calories
Fat	27 grams
Protein	31 grams
Carbohydrate	NONE

Appendix

7. Real Whipped Cream

Many people have forgotten what real whipped cream is. Once you try this, you will never go back to the artificial stuff. Have it plain or on Sugar-Free Jell-O.™

Ingredients	Amount
Heavy whipping cream	2 tablespoons
Liquid artificial sweetener	Optional, to taste

Instructions: Place cream and sweetener in a cool, deep bowl. Using an electric mixer with cool beaters, whip it until it doubles in size and thickens. Store any unused amounts in a closed refrigerator container.

	Alone	with Jell-O™
Energy	90 calories	92 calories
Fat	10 grams	10 grams
Protein	NONE	1 gram
Carbohydrate	NONE	NONE

Note: Use the Sugar-Free Jell-O™ you mix yourself. Pre-mixed cups have added carbohydrates. Avoid brands that have more ingredients than others. Use flavors that are marked 5 calories or less.

---

8. Real Cream Soda

Whether you want to increase the proportion of fat in a particular meal or just have a delicious beverage, try this real cream soda.

Ingredients	Amount
Flavored diet soda (cola, cream, or root beer)	Enough to fill a glass
Heavy cream	1 tablespoon
Ice cubes	as needed

Instructions: Place ice in the glass first, then add the cream. Next, pour in the soda, but avoid lemon flavor. Stir briefly as it froths. Drink up and enjoy

Energy	45 calories
Fat	5 grams
Protein	NONE
Carbohydrate	NONE

Fighting Covid-19, the Unequal Opportunity Killer

9. Chicken Mole

Mole, pronounced *mo-lay*, is a Mexican dish, which has many regional variations. It contains chocolate, ground nuts, chili pepper, other spices, and sweetener. This recipe does not claim authenticity but it is tasty. Vary it as you like. It works well with other dishes besides Chicken, too.

Ingredients	Amount
Chicken breast	½ portion, about 4 ounces
Olive oil	2 tablespoons
100% cocoa powder	1 teaspoon
Cinnamon	½ teaspoon, to taste
Liquid non-calorie sweetener	1 teaspoon, to taste
Hot pepper sauce	½ teaspoon, to taste
Natural peanut butter	1 teaspoon, to taste
Ground red pepper	½ teaspoon, to taste

Instructions: Cook chicken by sautéing it in oil in a frying pan. Lower heat to simmer and mix in other ingredients. Stir to mix as peanut butter softens. If needed, add a little water or MSG-free chicken broth to thin. Cover and simmer for a few minutes to allow flavors to mix. If you desire, you may add other ingredients, such as sliced mushrooms. You may also want to try this as a meat or chicken stir-fry, featuring cut-up leftovers and vegetables.

Energy	178 calories
Fat	18 grams
Protein	27 grams
Carbohydrate	2 grams

---

10. Creamy Curry Sauce

This simple sauce is a great way to balance the proportion of fat in meals, while adding taste. It goes with many foods. Try it on lightly steamed asparagus.

Ingredients	Amount
Real Mayonnaise	1 tablespoon
Curry Powder	about ½ teaspoon, to taste

Instructions: Mix the curry powder and mayonnaise thoroughly. Allow to stand a few minutes before using. If larger amounts are mixed, be sure to refrigerate.

Energy	99 calories
Fat	11 grams
Protein	NONE
Carbohydrate	NONE

Appendix

Supplements to consider

Don't skip over this section. A few easily available supplements may be valuable to you, but beware of expensive hoaxes. Have you heard about the magic herbal compound from a remote Pacific Island that grows in special volcanic soil? Neither have I, but this is the type of hoax found in late night infomercials, printed ads, and social media. Even worse than those hucksters are people you think are professionals but are trying to sell you their own various supplements. I suggest that you avoid claims made by those who recommend a supplement which you can only buy from them.

Fiber is an absolute necessity on this diet and is recommended for everyone. Your body will process the food found in this diet with very little waste, which results in smaller bowel movements. Your intestines stretched for the larger amounts you might have eaten before, so a smaller amount of waste goes nowhere until you gradually become constipated. Adding fiber to your diet from the beginning prevents this problem from happening. The most reliable supplement is *psyllium fiber*, available as *Sugar-Free Metamucil*® powder. People avoiding the aspartame sweetener should use an unflavored psyllium fiber instead. Fiber is not a laxative. Laxatives, such as Miralax® should be reserved for actual constipation. The right type of fiber can prevent such problems. Follow the label directions so that you experience a daily bowel movement without straining or discomfort. This consistent pattern will reduce the "transit time" of your waste and is associated with fewer gastrointestinal problems, including colon cancer. The good news is that if you are consistent, your body will gradually adjust to the smaller volume, so much so that eating today's larger portions will seem abnormal.

A daily multivitamin and mineral supplement is a safety net on any diet. Individual needs and food choices vary, putting dieters at risk of missing some important micronutrient. A daily multivitamin and mineral supplement may theoretically fill many of these gaps, although you should avoid chewable sugar-laden gummy vitamins. Recent revelations have shown that the actual distribution within any given multivitamin pill can be erratic, so stick to a major brand. If you believe you have a deficiency for a specific vitamin or mineral, add that as an individual pill!

Vitamin D is important for your immune system response, both to the pandemic and for many other issues. This is well-covered in Chapter 7. Follow those recommendations.

Fighting Covid-19, the Unequal Opportunity Killer

Zinc is a mineral that serves as a cofactor in more than 70 enzyme systems. A zinc deficiency can also weaken your immune response, so consider taking additional zinc. Supplements containing a combination of zinc, magnesium and calcium are available or it can be taken individually. Zinc deficiency Is difficult for your physician to evaluate, since mineral blood levels often do not reflect actual levels in your tissue.

Magnesium deficiency is found in one-fourth of diabetics and increases when dieting. One symptom for dieters is nighttime leg muscle cramping, another may be hair loss. These often respond quickly to a magnesium supplement. Again, this deficiency is difficult to evaluate through blood tests, since your blood level may not reflect your actual tissue level.

Potassium deficiency may be found combined with magnesium efficiency. Potassium deficiency may be caused if you are using a diuretic medication or "water pill," something your physician should be monitoring. Electrolyte imbalance from heat and the activity may also contribute to a low level. As with other minerals, blood level is not always an accurate indication of tissue level. When concentrated potassium is needed, it is often prescribed by your doctor. This can be difficult to take and very upsetting to the stomach. Less concentrated forms are found in balanced sugar-free sports drinks. Don't try the popular idea of eating bananas for potassium, they contain far more sugar than they do potassium. A balanced way to boost potassium is to exchange your table salt for a 50-50 mixture of iodized sodium chloride and potassium chloride, such as Morton Lite® Salt. These minerals are closely linked in your body. The idea that we generally use too much table salt was covered in Chapter 3 and discussed further below. Science has shown that most Americans generally receive too much **sodium** from processed foods, particularly when it is found in hidden MSG.

Iodine is another mineral that is is important for human life. It is needed for your thyroid to function properly. Today, many people are diagnosed with low thyroid output (hypothyroidism), which regulates much of your body's metabolism. Today, they are generally prescribed synthetic thyroid hormone replacement therapy. Although thyroid medication is inexpensive, it does not compensate for the underlying cause of iodine deficiency. It is difficult to evaluate iodine levels without a blood test combined with a 24-hour urine collection.

Iodine deficiency was recognized a century ago, when doctors realized that people living on either coast who regularly ate fresh ocean fish, a rich source of iodine, were less likely to have hypothyroidism than people

Appendix

living in the Midwest. Some people were prescribed Lugol's solution, an supplement still available over-the-counter. A more practical solution was to add iodine to everyone's diet by iodizing table salt. At that time, most people used table salt. The addition of potassium iodide to ordinary table salt largely reduced that then common problem. That simple solution worked so well that its purpose had been largely forgotten by the time the government began discouraging table salt use. **Blaming the imbalance of dietary sodium on ordinary salt protected the food industry by diverting attention away from the fact that almost all processed food today contain sodium from MSG**, whether open or hidden. As people eliminated table salt from their diet, they undid the benefit of having an adequate dietary source of iodine. If you have been diagnosed with hypothyroidism, discuss this with your physician.

Folate, also known as folic acid, is an important B vitamin. Both diabetics and people who are obese tend to be deficient. Low folate can cause many problems and dieters may notice hair loss. Some other issues can be anemia, heart disease and hypertension. Pregnant women are given extra folate to prevent neural tube defects in their children. Folate can be found naturally in green leafy vegetables. Your physician can easily check your blood level and will often check your Vitamin B12 level at the same time. Supplements are available without prescription.

Vitamin B_{12} is important for both blood forming and the nervous system. In severe cases, a lack of it may cause dementia, which may be reversible if discovered early. Deficiencies are usually found both in people who avoid red meat and those who do not absorb it well from their stomach. People following strict vegetarian diets should pay attention to getting enough Vitamin B_{12}. Although there is a condition where vitamin B_{12} cannot be absorbed in adequate amounts, today there are other causes. Stomach surgery for weight-loss can cause this problem, as can the use of common proton-pump inhibitors, which are drugs taken for gastric reflux, heartburn or indigestion. If this applies to you, ask your physician for a simple blood test. If there is an absorption problem, monthly injections were once were common. Today, non-prescription B_{12} is available in a sublingual form. Sublingual means you can let the supplement dissolve under your tongue, where it is absorbed directly into your blood, bypassing the problem.

Chromium is trace mineral which is a cofactor in maintaining glucose control. Although a lack of chromium has be shown to be a factor for developing diabetes in an animal model, it is not clear whether this is an important consideration in people. Some scientists advocate its use, in amounts of 1 mg or 1,000 mcg (micrograms) each day for diabetics. It is

Fighting Covid-19, the Unequal Opportunity Killer

found in over-the-counter as Chromium Picolinate. It appears to be safe and inexpensive, so it may be worth trying but it's value has not been established.

Carnitine is needed to burn fat. Most people receive an adequate supply in their diet, except those who avoid red meat. If you have difficulty initiating and maintaining fat burning, you might benefit from this supplement. It is sold in pharmacies as L-Carnitine.

DHEA or Dehydroepiandrosterone is normally made within the body to be turned into sex hormones. Exaggerated claims have been made by those profiting from its sale. Research has shown that it may be useful in decreasing abdominal fat, but it should be used cautiously and with your physician's knowledge, since it may help the body increase its level of testosterone in both men and women. That may increase energy level and sex drive for some while also decreasing depression, but it has drawbacks. People suffering from polycystic ovary disorder, heart disease, or surviving any form of cancer that is sensitive to hormones should avoid using it. Discuss this with you doctor.

Niacin is an important B vitamin. Most people get enough niacin in their diet to prevent niacin deficiency (pellagra). One type of niacin, nicotinic acid, can also improve cholesterol balance, but only in higher doses. It is inexpensive and available without a prescription, yet it can be more effective than prescribed statin drugs, without their drawback of muscle pain and damage. Nicotinic acid not only lowers bad cholesterol, it can simultaneously increase HDL good cholesterol! Although its value has been understood for decades, it is cheap and generic so it is not pushed like costly medications. Discuss this with your physician if you are interested in improving your cholesterol balance. People who should not take nicotinic acid include pregnant women and anyone with liver disease.

Only nicotinic acid has the cholesterol-lowering effect. The other forms of niacin (niacinamide and inositol hexaniotinate) will prevent classic niacin deficiency but not alter cholesterol balance. Look for the niacin bottle to either clearly state that it is nicotinic acid, or it has a label warning about a flush. The drawback of nicotinic acid is that shortly after it is taken blood vessels in your skin will open causing a red flush accompanied by an uncomfortable sensation of burning and itching which will last for several minutes. You must use it correctly to overcome this drawback. If started on niacin, find the smallest size that you can, typically 250 or 500 mg, breaking it into quarters and start on this small daily dose. Take a small 81 mg aspirin shortly before taking the niacin. You should barely feel the flush after doing

Appendix

this for several days, then slowly increase the amount as your body becomes accustomed to niacin. Gradually work your way up until you are taking a total of 1500 to 2000 mg a day without discomfort. Doing it this way, you should find the flushing to be barely noticeable. Slow-release niacin is also available, in an effort to reduce flushing, but that form can be irritating to your liver. Your physician should routinely check your liver as part of your annual blood chemistry.

Co-enzyme Q10 is a supplement needed if you have take a statin drug. A statin may rob your body this important coenzyme and lead to muscular problems. If you take a statin drug, consider this supplement as protection from potentially harm of the statin drug.

Avoid all products claiming to boost your metabolism to lose weight. Whether prescription or non-prescription, these are all variants on a theme and all pose the same dangers. They tend to increase the work of your heart and increase your blood pressure while burning more calories and reducing your appetite. Many of these dangerous drugs come on the market claiming complete safety, only to be restricted or pulled off the market later, after harming people. **That is not a new development. In the 1890s cocaine was a popular weight-loss prescription. Beginning in the 1930s, so was amphetamine!**

Avoiding chemical flavor enhancers

Chapters 10 and 11 discussed hidden flavor enhancers and finding them on labels. Food companies are often international, but when the sell product in the United States they take advantage of loopholes in our regulation in hiding what they would rather the public does not recognize. This makes avoiding these dangers an ongoing battle, needing you constant attention and vigilance. Here is an expanded list of names to watch for. **Be aware of the many names of hidden chemical flavor enhancers.**

Fighting Covid-19, the Unequal Opportunity Killer

Names or Words Often Associated with Chemical Flavor Enhancers

Certainly or Probably Contains MSG or a Similar Chemical

Autolyzed "anything"
Autolyzed plant protein
Autolyzed yeast
Calcium caseinate
Disodium inosinate
Disodium guanylate
DSG
DSI
Glutamate
Glutamic acid
HPP

HVP
Hydrolyzed "anything"
Hydrolyzed corn protein
Hydrolyzed soy protein
Hydrolyzed plant protein
Hydrolyzed vegetable protein
Monopotassium glutamate
Monosodium glutamate
Sodium caseinate
Textured protein
Vegetable broth

Other Items or Names Often Associated with Chemical Enhancers

Barley malt
Broth, stock or bouillon
Caramel flavoring or coloring
Carrageenan
Citric acid (when processed from corn)
Cornstarch
Dough conditioners
Fermented "anything"
Flavors, flavoring, seasonings, spice, extract, reaction flavors when are not given specific names
Flowing agents
Gelatin (except gelatin desserts)
Gums
Imitation or faux seafood and meat
"Krab" instead of crab

Lipolyzed butter fat
"Low" or "No-fat" items
Malted barley
Modified "anything"
Modified food starch
Natural chicken, beef, or pork flavoring
Pectin enzymes
Protease
Protease enzymes milk, whey-protein, whey, milk powder, dry milk solids, whey protein isolate or concentrate
Protein-fortified "anything"
Soy, wheat, rice, or oat protein
Soy sauce or extract
Soy-protein isolate or concentrate

or any ingredients that appear out of place for the food they are in!

Appendix

Deciding on Sweeteners

Sweeteners are the ingredients people ask about the most. If you desire to add sweetness, use saccharin in water, whenever it is practical. All forms of real sugar are sugar to your body. Some have different tastes, some raise your blood sugar level slightly faster; some sugars are created artificially by breaking down starches; many cost extra because they are from exotic sources. Some, such as high fructose corn syrup, may taste sweeter than others. It really doesn't matter, since they all can do the same harm.

In the last century and a half, humankind throughout the world has become so accustomed to the taste of these sugar-laden products that weaning from them seems difficult. Actually, most people will gradually lose their desire for hyper-sweetened products once they have been on a ketogenic diet for a while. Once the physical uplift from that jolt of rapidly rising blood sugar goes away, the psychological connection tying hyper-sweetened flavor to comfort will gradually decline.

In the interim, people prefer the sweetened taste they expect. That is the reason non-calorie sweeteners exist. Many people are frightened because non-calorie sweeteners are deemed artificial. True, most non-calorie sweeteners may not exist in that form in nature, but it is also true that much of the sugar in use today is equally artificial. Although actual sugar may come from natural sources, much of the sugar today is factory created. Starches in plant material have to be chemically extracted and modified to turn them into sugar. It really all becomes a matter of definition. When choosing a sweetened product, be careful when the front label states "*Made with Stevia*" or some similar ingredient. The front label tells you that it contains a particular ingredient but the ingredients list can show that it also contains other sweeteners, even sugar.

An industry myth is that using sugar substitutes makes you gain weight. That idea comes from bad science. If you interview people who use sugar substitutes, you would find that many are heavier. That is the reason they turned to sugar substitutes, not the cause of their being overweight. A few decades back, cigarette companies advertised that certain brands were good for your lungs. This was the same type of science.

Restaurants in the United States provide paper packets of sugar or sweeteners for beverages. Each packet should provide about the same degree of sweetness as a teaspoon of sugar. In Europe, you bring your own

Fighting Covid-19, the Unequal Opportunity Killer

non-calorie sweeteners. Stores sell small dispensers that contain tablets, which are a mixture of sweetening chemicals.

Pure artificial sweeteners are stronger than the same amount of sugar. When artificial sweeteners were first used in the late 19th-century, it was in place of sugar in processed foods to lower their cost. That was considered adulteration or fraud and highly controversial. The high strength of sweeteners became a problem when measuring tiny individual dosages, for people who were trying to avoid sugar. The first solution was to put the sweetener in a pill, but those early pills were difficult to dissolve. That problem was "solved" by combining the sweetener with a "flowing agent," resulting in the powdered products we see today. However, the original flowing agent was actually sugar!

Industry has used an FDA loophole, which still exists today. **Products containing less than 5 calories are allowed to be labeled "zero calories."** Today, different products contain various flowing agents, but that packet of sweetener may contain "only" about one fourth the calories of a teaspoon of sugar but that is far from "sugar free." The safest flowing agent is water. That is why I always recommend a liquid form when purchasing sugar substitutes for home use.

Saccharin is the original sugar substitute, produced since the late 19th-century. It is also the most misunderstood. It has never been shown to produce any harm or disease in people. The only negative aspect of saccharin is that some people sense a bitter taste when the solid form is used in high doses. In the past, there were suspicions because saccharin was produced from chemical found in coal tar. At extremely high doses, thousands of times the normal level, it increased the chance of cancers in laboratory rats. Further research showed that was not true for humans; it applied only to rats because of certain unique chemistry. Saccharin became cheap and generic, so chemical companies attacked it when they developed more profitable substitutes. There was an attempt in the 1970s to ban saccharin and allow a rival sweetener, cyclamate, to dominate the market in the United States. Then potential problems with cyclamate surfaced, and instead, it was cyclamate that was banned in the United States. Canada moved faster then the United States and had already banned saccharin by that time. This resulted in the brand names associated with yellow and pink packets to sell one product in the United States under their color-code scheme and sell just the opposite in Canada. As better science cleared saccharin of any problems, Canada relented and has once again approved saccharin in their country. In the United States, saccharin is also available in

Appendix

a liquid form.

Aspartame has been the most popular artificial sweetener in the United States for many years. It is found in most diet drinks and took over once cyclamate was banned. It should be used with caution, since there is an FDA-set upper limit on its recommended use. It quickly found its way into diet sodas because of a sweet taste without a bitter aftertaste. Problems have been reported, yet well-funded studies by the drug and chemical industries studies fail to show any problems, except for the restriction that people who have PKU (phenylketonuria, a genetic defect that makes them sensitive to phenylalanine) should never use aspartame.

It is likely that problems are most common in a subset of people. Some people complain they develop headaches, perhaps from formaldehyde associated with aspartame. It may counteract psychiatric drugs, such as anti-depressants People who are sensitive stop using it so they do not show up in research on the general population. There also might be a crossover with other sensitivities, since some people who have complaints using aspartame also report they are sensitive to MSG. Aspartame is also sensitive to heat and should never be used in cooking or baking. During the Persian Gulf War, diet soda was shipped to warehouses in the desert where the internal temperature was extreme. Aspartame broke down and made the drinks unusable and dangerous. Since then, aspartame-sweetened diet drinks have a printed "use by date". One interesting note is that the Commissioner of the FDA left that agency a few months after approving aspartame as an ingredient in soda. He then accepted a position at a firm used by the company that developed aspartame. Fortunately, some newer diet drinks are beginning to be made with other sweeteners.

Cyclamate became popular in the United States in the 1970s but was withdrawn from the market due to unfavorable studies. Although those studies have since been questioned, it remains banned in the United States while it is used in many other countries.

Sucralose is actually made by modifying the table sugar sucrose so that it is not absorbed by the body. It is popular in baking and other cooking because of its consistency. It is difficult to calculate its true carbohydrate load, since it is used with a flowing agent. Under FDA regulations they claim it is zero calories because the label refers to a small teaspoon serving. In contradiction, that same label may contain recipes calling for its use by the cupful! Use it in baking if this is your only choice but try to limit the amount by mixing with true non-calorie sweeteners. Be cautious and always read the label carefully, since some sucralose products mix it with regular sugar.

Fighting Covid-19, the Unequal Opportunity Killer

Acesulfame is used as an ingredient in many manufactured and baked goods. Because of a slight bitter aftertaste it is often used in combination with other sweeteners and not as a stand-alone product.

Stevia started out as the only truly natural sweetener, found in nature without chemical processing. It has been in use for millennia by indigenous people of South America. It is not perfect, since some people may find it sweeter than others, and it can have a bitter aftertaste from other chemicals in the stevia leaf. It is fairly new in the United States, originally marketed using the exemption for nutritional products. Using it as an ingredient in processed food required costly testing and FDA approval. That process was only financially worthwhile if it could be patented, so a producer went to the trouble of chemically modifying stevia just for that reason. Today, two types of stevia exist, the natural form and the chemically altered version. Stevia is also available as a liquid sweetener.

Sugar alcohols are a group of unusual chemicals. They do not contain the intoxicant alcohol. Look for ingredient names ending in "ol". On one hand, they chemically resemble sugar and signal your taste buds that they are real sugar. On the other hand, they have what chemists call an alcohol group, **OH**, which consists of an atom of oxygen attached to an atom of hydrogen. This extra little tail prevents them from being absorbed from your gastrointestinal tract Unfortunately, gas-producing bacteria in your gastrointestinal tract like sugar alcohol. Eat too much and they multiply, producing gas, cramping, and diarrhea. Most people can tolerate sugar alcohol in small amounts, such as in sugar-free chewing gum. However, low carbohydrate ice cream may be more of a temptation to overeat. As these bacteria feast on the sugar alcohol, it breaks it in a way that frees some remaining sugar, that can be absorbed and raise blood sugar. Sugar alcohols can be a safe product when used in moderation but cause problems when their use is overdone.

The Fats You Eat

Fat is the most efficient way to store nutritional energy. since a gram of fat contains 9 calories of energy. Fats are described by many characteristics but the common perception of what is good or bad has been influenced by industry. Here are a few thoughts to help you choose your dietary fat.

1. **Trans fat should always be avoided.** The main source of trans

Appendix

fat is hydrogenation, which is why they are also called **hydrogenated fats**. The purpose of hydrogenation is to take inexpensive vegetable fat and give it more body to resemble thicker, more expensive fat. That is how margarine is produced to resemble butter. Hydrogenation is an industrial process invented in the 19th century to change the way the atoms in a molecule of fat bind to each other. In nature, fats are created in a step-by-step process, resulting in bonds between atoms that create a natural shape. In hydrogenation, these bonds are created on a mass scale, and produce two very different molecules, as if one were a mirror image of another. Since hydrogenated fats contain substantial amounts of unnatural backwards molecules or trans fats, this is not how nature intended it. No matter how hard they try to make margarine look like butter, it is still margarine. *Avoid any food where you find the word hydrogenated in the ingredients.*

2. **Your gallbladder is an important part of your digestive system.** To digest most fats, they are first broken down by bile salts created in your liver. Bile salts are produced slowly and are stored in your gallbladder. If you eat a fatty meal, your gallbladder squirts out enough bile salt for your fats to be digested. If you eat very little fat, these bile salts can begin stagnate and crystallize, forming small solid particles, which can grow into stones. Then, when you use your gall bladder, those stones can get stuck causing inflammation and pain. One contradiction here, eating a fatty meal may cause the gallbladder attack but it was not eating fat that caused the stagnation, which formed the gallstones. If you have gallstones or sand-like sludge in you gallbladder, there is a medication that can slowly dissolve them over several months and may prevent an attack.

If you have an acute gallbladder attack, surgically removing your gallbladder is the usual therapy. Gallbladder attacks may occur hours after eating a fatty meal. They are characterized by severe acute right-sided abdominal pain just below the rib cage and often radiating to the back. Often, the person suffering this severe pain visits the emergency room late at night and has surgery the next morning. Other people may go for years carrying gallstones or sludge in their gallbladder without an acute attack, but have problems digesting fat. They may have cramping and loose, light-colored bowel movements when they eat fat. They could be candidates for medical treatment rather than surgery, for once their gallbladder is removed, their digestion will never be the same. Their liver will still produce the needed bile salts but the loss of their storage reserve means that eating large amounts of fat at one time can be a problem.

3. **Coconut oil and MCT oil are special.** These products can help

Fighting Covid-19, the Unequal Opportunity Killer

those who have had their gallbladder removed. Coconut oil is a natural source of a special fat that can be digested without the help of bile salt. This is called a medium-chain triglyceride or MCT and it is the right size to be absorbed without help from bile salts. People who have had their gall bladder removed can benefit from this, using it as a substitute for other fat. Coconut oil is unattractive, white, and thick at room temperature, while MCT oil is coconut oil that has been modified to make it clear and liquid. Neither is particularly tasty. Coconut oil recently became a fad, with some ketogenic diet proponents recommending that everyone start their day with a shot of it in their coffee. This practice can help those who have difficulty digesting fat, but is not needed for those without problems. Try some real cream in your coffee, instead.

4. **Dietary cholesterol is not your enemy.** Your body makes its own cholesterol for good reason, since cholesterol is an important building block. An imbalance of your body's cholesterol can be an important marker for metabolic problems. Serum cholesterol that is too low will cause a failure of normal sexual hormones and is associated with depression and suicide. Levels that seem too high should be evaluated for balance between your different types of cholesterol. The metabolic practices described in this book can reverse those imbalances.

5. **A balance of different types of fat is good for you.** Olive oil is a very healthy source of monounsaturated fat. Fish oils are high in Omega-3 fatty acids but are much better when they come from fish than from a capsule. Fish with dark flesh is higher in healthy fish oil than fish that is white. Saturated fats are natural in animal products. Butter, eggs, cheese and cream are good sources. The fear about saturated fat was overdone since your body needs it to make cholesterol, which is necessary for a normal healthy life. Saturated fat also helps create increase your HDL, the "good cholesterol". **Think balance, not demonization.**

Appendix

Recipe Worksheet

Recipe for _____

Number of servings _____

Ingredient & Amount	F gm 9	P gm 4	C gm 4	calories
1				
2				
3				
4				
5				
6				
7				
8				
9				
10				
Totals per recipe add columns	grams	grams	grams	calories
Divide the above line by the number of servings in this recipe.				
Amounts per Serving	grams	grams	grams	calories

Cooking instructions & comments:

This worksheet is for developing your own recipes or checking recipes you find elsewhere. As you list each ingredient and amount, fill in the grams for fat, protein, and carbohydrate. Total these amounts, then divide these results by the number of servings to determine the grams per serving.

About the Author

Irving Cohen, M.D., M.P.H. is a physician who has dedicated his medical career to the prevention of disease, focusing on early detection and interventions to prevent more serious disease outcomes later. He left a successful computer career to help people struggling with disease. Following medical school, he initially trained in Internal Medicine but recognized that conventional medical practice focused on treating illness that might have been preventable. He then turned his attention to the medical specialty of Preventive Medicine. Dr. Cohen trained in Preventive Medicine and Public Health at the Johns Hopkins University, Bloomberg School of Public Health. He served there as a Resident Physician and then as Chief Resident of Preventive Medicine. He has been Board-Certified in Preventive Medicine and Public Health by the American Board of Preventive Medicine for 35 years and is a Fellow of the American College of Preventive Medicine.

Dr. Cohen has served in private practice and government service, in public health and clinical medicine. He was Deputy Director of the New York State Research Institute on Addiction. He has held faculty appointments at the State University of New York at Buffalo School of Medicine, the University of Kansas School of Medicine and the Karl Menninger School of Psychiatry and Mental Health Sciences.

After he thought he had retired, he became interested in the emerging epidemics of overweight, obesity, and diabetes. Developing an improved way to evaluate the efficacy of weight-loss methods and studying effective historical techniques led him to develop programs for weight-loss and diabetes control. He has made presentations about these topics at medical scientific forums in the United States and Canada and is the author of books on losing weight and reversing diabetes.

When the Covid-19 epidemic struck the world, he recognized that the differential risk of serious illness and death was modifiable. He has written this book to alert the public that they are not helpless, whether their increased risk is associated with age, race, or pre-existing chronic illness.